NATIONAL   Scienc
ACADEMIES   Engin
            Medici

Data Integration in Learning Health Care Systems for Traumatic Brain Injury

Tamara Haag, Chanel Matney, and
Katherine Bowman, *Rapporteurs*

Forum on Traumatic Brain Injury

Board on Health Sciences Policy

Health and Medicine Division

Proceedings of a Workshop

NATIONAL ACADEMIES PRESS 500 Fifth Street, NW Washington, DC 20001

This activity was supported by contracts and grants between the National Academy of Sciences and Abbott Laboratories; AARP; Brain Scope, Inc.; Department of Defense (contract W81XWH22C0033); Department of Veterans Affairs (contract 36C24E22P0005); National Highway Traffic Safety Administration; National Institute on Disability, Independent Living, and Rehabilitation Research (contract 140D0423C0099 through the Department of the Interior); National Institutes of Health (contract HHSN263201800029I, task order 75N98022F00001); Neurotrauma Sciences; American Academy of Nursing; American Academy of Physical Medicine and Rehabilitation; American Association of Neurological Surgeons; American College of Surgeons; American Physical Therapy Association; Brain Injury Association of America; Concussion Legacy Foundation;; Emergency Nurses Association; National Association of Emergency Medical Technicians; National Association of State Head Injury Administrators; and National College Athletic Association. Any opinions, findings, conclusions, or recommendations expressed in this publication do not necessarily reflect the views of any organization or agency that provided support for the project.

International Standard Book Number-13: 978-0-309-71744-1
International Standard Book Number-10: 0-309-71744-2
Digital Object Identifier: https://doi.org/10.17226/27653

This publication is available from the National Academies Press, 500 Fifth Street, NW, Keck 360, Washington, DC 20001; (800) 624-6242 or (202) 334-3313; http://www.nap.edu.

Suggested citation: National Academies of Sciences, Engineering, and Medicine. 2024. *Data integration in learning health care systems for traumatic brain injury: Proceedings of a workshop.* Washington, DC: The National Academies Press. https://doi.org/10.17226/27653.

The **National Academy of Sciences** was established in 1863 by an Act of Congress, signed by President Lincoln, as a private, nongovernmental institution to advise the nation on issues related to science and technology. Members are elected by their peers for outstanding contributions to research. Dr. Marcia McNutt is president.

The **National Academy of Engineering** was established in 1964 under the charter of the National Academy of Sciences to bring the practices of engineering to advising the nation. Members are elected by their peers for extraordinary contributions to engineering. Dr. John L. Anderson is president.

The **National Academy of Medicine** (formerly the Institute of Medicine) was established in 1970 under the charter of the National Academy of Sciences to advise the nation on medical and health issues. Members are elected by their peers for distinguished contributions to medicine and health. Dr. Victor J. Dzau is president.

The three Academies work together as the **National Academies of Sciences, Engineering, and Medicine** to provide independent, objective analysis and advice to the nation and conduct other activities to solve complex problems and inform public policy decisions. The National Academies also encourage education and research, recognize outstanding contributions to knowledge, and increase public understanding in matters of science, engineering, and medicine.

Learn more about the National Academies of Sciences, Engineering, and Medicine at **www.nationalacademies.org**.

Consensus Study Reports published by the National Academies of Sciences, Engineering, and Medicine document the evidence-based consensus on the study's statement of task by an authoring committee of experts. Reports typically include findings, conclusions, and recommendations based on information gathered by the committee and the committee's deliberations. Each report has been subjected to a rigorous and independent peer-review process and it represents the position of the National Academies on the statement of task.

Proceedings published by the National Academies of Sciences, Engineering, and Medicine chronicle the presentations and discussions at a workshop, symposium, or other event convened by the National Academies. The statements and opinions contained in proceedings are those of the participants and are not endorsed by other participants, the planning committee, or the National Academies.

Rapid Expert Consultations published by the National Academies of Sciences, Engineering, and Medicine are authored by subject-matter experts on narrowly focused topics that can be supported by a body of evidence. The discussions contained in rapid expert consultations are considered those of the authors and do not contain policy recommendations. Rapid expert consultations are reviewed by the institution before release.

For information about other products and activities of the National Academies, please visit www.nationalacademies.org/about/whatwedo.

PLANNING COMMITTEE[1]

CORINNE PEEK-ASA (*Chair*), Vice Chancellor for Research and Professor of Epidemiology, University of California, San Diego

DAVID GOLDSTEIN, Senior Advisor, Office of the Assistant Secretary for Health, Department of Health and Human Services

ODETTE HARRIS, Paralyzed Veterans of America Professor of Spinal Cord Injury Medicine, Professor and Vice Chair, Diversity, Department of Neurosurgery, Stanford University School of Medicine, and Deputy Chief of Staff, Rehabilitation, Veterans Affairs Palo Alto Health Care System

MICHAEL HUERTA, Acting Deputy Director for Operations and Innovation, National Library of Medicine, National Institutes of Health

MONIQUE PAPPADIS, Associate Professor, Department of Population Health and Health Disparities, University of Texas Medical Branch at Galveston

NSINI UMOH, Program Director, Division of Neuroscience, National Institute of Neurological Disorders and Stroke, National Institutes of Health

REBECCAH WOLFKIEL, Executive Director, National Association of State Injury Administrators

KRISTINE YAFFE, Scola Endowed Chair, Vice Chair, and Professor, Departments of Psychiatry, Neurology, and Epidemiology, University of California, San Francisco

Health and Medicine Division Staff

KATHERINE BOWMAN, Senior Program Officer, Board on Health Sciences Policy

CHANEL MATNEY, Program Officer, Board on Health Sciences Policy

GAYATRI SOMAIYA, Senior Program Assistant, Board on Health Sciences Policy

CLARE STROUD, Senior Director, Board on Health Sciences Policy

Consultants

TAMARA HAAG, Science Writer, Doxastic
ANNA NICHOLSON, Founder and Lead Writer, Doxastic

---

[1] The National Academies of Sciences, Engineering, and Medicine's planning committees are solely responsible for organizing the workshop, identifying topics, and choosing speakers. The responsibility for the published Proceedings of a Workshop rests with the workshop rapporteurs and the institution.

FORUM ON TRAUMATIC BRAIN INJURY[1]

DONALD BERWICK (*Cochair*), Institute for Healthcare Improvement
CORINNE PEEK-ASA (*Cochair*), University of California, San Diego
JOE BONNER, Eunice Kennedy Shriver National Institute of Child Health
and Human Development
JOE BRENNAN, Avalon Action Alliance
JAVIER CÁRDENAS, West Virginia University and American Academy of
Neurology
JOHN CORRIGAN, Ohio State University and Brain Injury Association of
America
JILL DAUGHERTY, Centers for Disease Control and Prevention
RAMON DIAZ-ARRASTIA, University of Pennsylvania Perelman School
of Medicine
E. WESLEY ELY, Vanderbilt University Medical Center
BRUCE EVANS, Upper Pine River Fire Protection District and National
Association of Emergency Medical Technicians
JONATHAN FISHER, American College of Emergency Physicians
STEVEN FLANAGAN, New York University Grossman School
of Medicine and American Academy of Physical Medicine and
Rehabilitation
BRIAN HAINLINE, National Collegiate Athletic Association
ODETTE HARRIS, Stanford University School of Medicine and VA Palo
Alto Health Care System
RICHARD HODES, National Institute on Aging
STUART HOFFMAN, Department of Veterans Affairs
JAMES KELLY, University of Colorado Anschutz Medical Campus
FREDERICK KORLEY, University of Michigan
WALTER KOROSHETZ, National Institute of Neurological Disorders
and Stroke
KATHY LEE, Department of Defense
RACHEL LAZARUS, AARP
D. CARL LONG, NeuroTrama Sciences, LLC
TARA JO MANAL, American Physical Therapy Association
GEOFFREY MANLEY, University of California, San Francisco, and
Zuckerberg San Francisco General Hospital
LUCA MARINELLI, GE Research
CHRISTINA L. MASTER, University of Pennsylvania Perelman School
of Medicine and Children's Hospital of Philadelphia

---

[1] The National Academies of Sciences, Engineering, and Medicine's forums and roundtables
do not issue, review, or approve individual documents. The responsibility for the published
Proceedings of a Workshop rests with the workshop rapporteurs and the institution.

BETH McQUISTON, Abbott Laboratories

CATE MILLER, National Institute on Disability, Independent Living, and Rehabilitation Research

CHRIS NOWINSKI, Concussion Legacy Foundation

KAREN O'CONNELL, Northern Kentucky University School of Nursing and Emergency Nurses Association

TESSIE OCTOBER, Eunice Kennedy Shriver National Institute of Child Health and Human Development

DAVID OKONKWO, University of Pittsburgh School of Medicine

TOLU O. OYESANYA, Duke University School of Nursing

MAYUR B. PATEL, Vanderbilt University Medical Center and American College of Surgeons Committee on Trauma

LESLIE PRICHEP, BrainScope Company, Inc.

TERRY RAUCH, Department of Defense

JOEL SCHOLTEN, Department of Veterans Affairs

SHELLY TIMMONS, Indiana University School of Medicine and American Association of Neurological Surgeons

GAMUNU WIJETUNGE, National Highway Traffic Safety Administration

REBECCAH WOLFKIEL, National Association of State Head Injury Administrators

KRISTINE YAFFE, University of California, San Francisco

Forum Staff

KATHERINE BOWMAN, Forum Director

CHANEL MATNEY, Program Officer

GAYATRI SOMAIYA, Senior Program Assistant

CHRISTIE BELL, Finance Business Partner

CLARE STROUD, Senior Director, Board on Health Sciences Policy

Reviewers

This Proceedings of a Workshop was reviewed in draft form by individuals chosen for their diverse perspectives and technical expertise. The purpose of this independent review is to provide candid and critical comments that will assist the National Academies of Sciences, Engineering, and Medicine in making each published proceedings as sound as possible and to ensure that it meets the institutional standards for quality, objectivity, evidence, and responsiveness to the charge. The review comments and draft manuscript remain confidential to protect the integrity of the process.

We thank the following individuals for their review of this proceedings:

JEANNE M. HOFFMAN, University of Washington
EDWIN LOMOTAN, Agency for Healthcare Research and Quality
MONICA VAVILALA, University of Washington

Although the reviewers listed above provided many constructive comments and suggestions, they were not asked to endorse the content of the proceedings, nor did they see the final draft before its release. The review of this proceedings was overseen by **CHRISTOPHER FORREST,** Children's Hospital of Philadelphia. He was responsible for making certain that an independent examination of this proceedings was carried out in accordance with standards of the National Academies and that all review comments were carefully considered. Responsibility for the final content rests entirely with the rapporteurs and the National Academies. We also thank staff member **MEREDITH YOUNG** for reading and providing helpful comments on this manuscript.

Contents

Box and Figures

Acronyms and Abbreviations

ACL	Administration on Community Living
AHRQ	Agency for Healthcare Research and Quality
AI	artificial intelligence
BARDA	Biomedical Advanced Research and Development Authority
BIA-NE	Brain Injury Alliance of Nebraska
BISC	Brain Injury Services Coordination
BRFSS	Behavioral Risk Factor Surveillance System
CARE4TBI	Comparing Treatment Approaches to Promote Inpatient Rehabilitation Effectiveness for TBI
CDC	Centers for Disease Control and Prevention
CENTER-TBI	Collaborative European Neurotrauma Effectiveness Research in TBI
CMMI	Center for Medicare and Medicaid Innovation
CMS	Centers for Medicare and Medicaid Services
CT	computerized tomography
CVD	cardiovascular disease
DARS	Department for Aging and Rehabilitative Services
DoD	Department of Defense
ED	emergency department
EHR	electronic health record

EMS   emergency medical services

FDA   U.S. Food and Drug Administration

GCS   Glasgow Coma Scale
GOSE   Glasgow Outcome Scale-Extended

ICD   International Classification of Diseases
IOM   Institute of Medicine
IT   information technology

LHS   learning health system
LIMBIC-CENC   Long-term Impact of Military-relevant Brain Injury
              Consortium—Chronic Effects of Neurotrauma
              Consortium

MOS   military occupational specialty

NAM   National Academy of Medicine
NASHIA   National Association of State Head Injury Administrators
NCSS   National Concussion Surveillance System
NIDILRR   National Institute on Disability, Independent Living, and
              Rehabilitation Research
NINDS   National Institute of Neurological Disorders and Stroke
NYU   New York University

OBISS   Online Brain Injury Screening and Support System
OR   operating room
OSU   Ohio State University
OSU TBI-ID   Ohio State University TBI Identification Method

PCP   primary care physician
PE   pulmonary emboli
PSC   Polytrauma Systems of Care
PTSD   post-traumatic stress disorder

RCT   randomized controlled trial

TBI   traumatic brain injury
TBICoE   Traumatic Brain Injury Center of Excellence
TED   TBI Endpoint Development
TRACK-TBI   Transforming Research and Clinical Knowledge in
              Traumatic Brain Injury

TRACTS   Translational Research Center for TBI and Stress
                Disorders

VA   Department of Veterans Affairs
VCU   Virginia Commonwealth University
VDH   Virginia Department of Health

1

Introduction[1]

Traumatic brain injury (TBI), in which an external force causes a disruption to normal brain physiology or function, affects millions of Americans each year. "Causes as diverse as falls, sports injuries, vehicle collisions, intimate partner violence, and military incidents can result in such injuries across a spectrum of severity and among every age group" (NASEM, 2022, p. 15) with symptoms that can be debilitating, long-lasting, and carry physical, cognitive, emotional, social, behavioral, and financial ramifications. The heterogeneity of TBI makes care and research challenging. The true prevalence of TBI is also not fully understood, given that most surveillance data come from hospital and patient health records, and many people who experience TBI, particularly at the milder end of the severity spectrum, do not seek hospital care. Individuals who do seek medical care often encounter challenges in navigating the stages of treatment and recovery after discharge from acute care. As several speakers noted during the workshop, the fragmented nature of the U.S. health care system and its siloed databases contribute to challenges in the patient experience and to knowledge gaps about TBI prevalence, comorbidities, risk factors, and longer-term outcomes. Learning health systems (LHSs) refer to research-partnered care networks that analyze data from patient care and other sources and use

---

[1] The planning committee's role was limited to planning the workshop, and the Proceedings of a Workshop was prepared by the workshop rapporteurs as a factual summary of what occurred at the workshop. Statements, recommendations, and opinions expressed are those of individual presenters and participants and are not necessarily endorsed or verified by the National Academies of Sciences, Engineering, and Medicine, and they should not be construed as reflecting any group consensus.

those insights to continuously improve their health services. Transforming TBI health systems and research networks into LHSs offers opportunities to expand the TBI knowledge base, accelerate advances in care, and address patient barriers to accessing effective treatment.

INTEGRATING THE LEARNING HEALTH SYSTEM CONCEPT AND THE TRAUMATIC BRAIN INJURY ROAD MAP

Odette Harris, professor of neurosurgery at Stanford University and deputy chief of staff for rehabilitation at the Veterans Affairs Palo Alto Health Care System, provided an overview of the development of the LHS concept and how this concept intersects with TBI needs and opportunities to advance research and improve care and recovery. In 2006, the Institute of Medicine convened the Roundtable on Evidence-Based Medicine in an effort to transform how evidence of clinical effectiveness is generated (IOM, 2007). The development of the LHS framework was born from that effort. The roundtable established the following priorities:

- Commitment to the right health care for each person;
- Putting the best evidence into practice;
- Establishing the effectiveness, efficiency, and safety of medical care delivered;
- Building constant measurement into our health care investments;
- Establishment of health care data as a public good;
- Shared responsibility distributed equitably across stakeholders, both public and private;
- Collaborative stakeholder involvement in setting priorities;
- Transparency in the execution of activities and reporting of results; and
- Subjugation of individual political or stakeholder perspectives in favor of the common good.

The roundtable focused on three dimensions of the challenge of creating a system that embodies these priorities: (1) fostering progress towards a long-term vision of an LHS, (2) advancing the discussion and activities necessary to meet the near-term need for expanded capacity to generate evidence to support medical care that is maximally effective and has the greatest value, and (3) improving a public understanding of the nature of evidence-based medicine. Although fully achieving these priorities would be impractical for all interventions, Harris said, discussions during a 2006 workshop and subsequent learning health system activities explored why "[t]he nation needs a healthcare system that learns" (IOM, 2007, p. 3).

The 2006 roundtable workshop highlighted challenges, uncertainties, and the compelling need for change, Harris continued. Aspects identified by workshop speakers within the need for change included adaptation to the pace of change, stronger synchrony of efforts, a culture of shared responsibility, a new clinical research paradigm, public engagement, incentives aligned for practice-based evidence, and leadership (IOM, 2007). Efforts to realize these goals included publication of *The Learning Health System Series*, which features numerous volumes on various LHS components.[2] Volume topics of particular relevance to this workshop include data utility, data quality, evidence, effectiveness research, digital platforms, and research and practice integration. Harris also underscored the importance of emphasizing effectiveness research rather than only efficacy research to understand results in real-world settings.

In 2020, the National Academies convened the Committee on Accelerating Progress in Traumatic Brain Injury Research and Care to develop a report that identifies major barriers and knowledge gaps impeding progress, highlights opportunities for collaborative action, and provides a road map to guide the TBI field, said Harris. The 18-member committee representing diverse disciplines used data from a literature review, public workshop and webinar sessions, and input from over 50 stakeholders in crafting the consensus report *Traumatic Brain Injury: A Roadmap for Accelerating Progress* (NASEM, 2022). The report considered the multiple stages of care after TBI: recognition, acute care, classification, rehabilitation, follow up, and recovery and reintegration (see Figure 1-1).

Recognition involves awareness of the signs and symptoms of TBI to properly identify individuals in need of medical treatment. Acute care provides the medical interventions needed to stabilize an individual after a TBI and mitigate ongoing damage resulting from the injury. Classification assesses the nature and severity of a TBI to inform diagnosis, prognosis, treatment, and reassessment as the condition evolves. Harris emphasized that classification is not a static diagnosis or assessment. To address the whole person, she said that rehabilitation interventions should be designed to improve physical, cognitive, and psychosocial functions and quality of life. Follow up involves continued engagement with the care system to identify and address ongoing and emerging needs, including provision of community-based support services. She also emphasized that follow up must be continuous and ongoing. Recovery and reintegration aim for recovery of function to the greatest extent possible, including return to family, community, work, or school.

---

[2] More information about *The Learning Health System Series*, including links to the various volumes, is available at https://nam.edu/programs/value-science-driven-health-care/learning-health-system-series/ (accessed December 12, 2023).

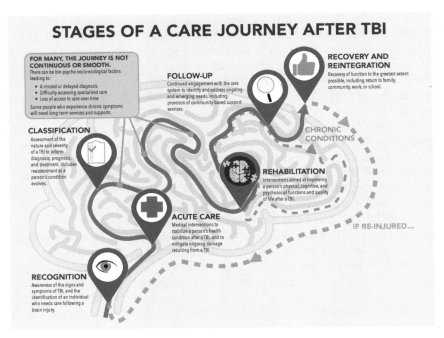

FIGURE 1-1 Stages of a care journey after TBI.
SOURCE: Presented by Odette Harris, October 12, 2023. NASEM, 2022.

As recognized in the report, navigating these stages is often not a continuous or smooth process, and biological, psychological, social, and ecological (bio-psycho-socio-ecological) factors can lead to missed or delayed diagnoses, difficulty accessing specialized care, and loss of access to care over time. Some individuals with TBI experience chronic symptoms and require long-term services and supports. Furthermore, re-injury can cause a person to restart the cycle-of-care stages, requiring consideration of the re-injury effects and stage-integration implications on a patient.

Harris highlighted several additional takeaways from the report:

- TBI is not an isolated, acute event and needs to be understood and managed as a condition influenced by numerous factors that can have long-term effects.
- An updated and more precise TBI classification system is needed to guide patient care and inform research.
- The United States lacks a comprehensive framework for the full continuum of care needed for individuals with TBI.

- An effective care system needs to anticipate, respond, and learn in a coordinated fashion.
- Progress has been made in TBI understanding and care, and opportunities for collaborative action could advance TBI awareness, prevention, treatment, and research (NASEM, 2022).

To help make progress in these and other areas, the report recommends better integrating TBI systems of care and TBI research into LHSs. Harris emphasized that these goals are aligned with the LHS core principles discussed at the 2006 IOM roundtable workshop, which explored how an LHS can be safe, effective, equitable, efficient, accessible, measurable, transparent, secure, and adaptive (described further in Chapter 2).

Following publication of the TBI *Roadmap* report, the National Academies established the ongoing Forum on Traumatic Brain Injury, the convener of this workshop, to advance the implementation of the report's recommendations and foster continued progress and innovation in TBI prevention, care, and recovery.[3] This workshop was designed to bring together lessons from the TBI report and LHS principles to explore how LHS practices can be operationalized to integrate knowledge and advance TBI care and research. Ultimately, Harris concluded, an improved system of TBI care and research stands to aid in providing patients and families with more effective services.

WORKSHOP OBJECTIVES

Fragmented and siloed TBI treatment and data undercut the current health system's ability to learn and improve (NASEM, 2022). LHSs are important contributors to progress in TBI, where much remains to be understood about prevalence, outcomes, and effective interventions. Achieving an integrated TBI system involves thorough surveillance efforts, standardization of patient-level data collection, and analysis of longitudinal data. To better understand the development of such a system, the Forum on Traumatic Brain Injury hosted a 1-day public workshop—Data Integration in Learning Health Care Systems for Traumatic Brain Injury—to explore needs, practices, and models for LHSs in the TBI field. Discussions did not focus on a specific type of TBI or sub-population that experiences it; rather, sessions aimed to introduce LHS concepts and illustrate their relevance to systems of care and research for this condition. The workshop, which was held virtually and in person on October 12, 2023, featured invited presentations and discussions to accomplish the following:

---

[3] Information about the forum and its activities is available at https://www.nationalacademies.org/our-work/traumatic-brain-injury-forum (accessed January 3, 2024).

- Explore the variables affecting how TBI patient data are collected, standardized, harmonized, accessed, and analyzed—and the LHS implications for TBI care and research.
- Discuss a vision for how enhanced TBI data integration in LHSs could improve care and advance clinical and epidemiological research.
- Consider key questions and priority use cases that could be explored through integrated patient record databases and TBI registries.
- Spotlight ongoing efforts towards building integrated research platforms and datasets for TBI.

ORGANIZATION OF THE PROCEEDINGS OF THE WORKSHOP

This proceedings summarizes the presentations and discussions from the workshop Data Integration in Learning Health Care Systems for Traumatic Brain Injury. The workshop highlighted selected opportunities, challenges, and strategies for fostering learning health systems, moving from the LHS concept and its applicability to unmet TBI care and research needs to the types of data, infrastructure, and partnerships needed to establish such systems. It featured examples of LHSs being created by health care organizations, federal agencies, and research networks, and illustrated how enhanced data integration and analysis could support learning and improvement. The workshop thus aimed to introduce how LHSs can help address unmet priorities and inform further efforts in this area but did not aim to cover all aspects comprehensively.

Following Chapter 1—which introduces the LHS framework and its relevance to advancing TBI care and research—Chapter 2 provides a personal account of the lived experienced of TBI, including effects of the condition, difficulty in navigating care systems, and barriers in accessing effective treatment. The chapter highlights the challenges that arise from fragmented and uncoordinated care and underscores the benefit of health information systems that enable provider collaboration and improve the patient navigation experience. Chapter 3 outlines the development of the LHS concept, the definition and core principles of an LHS, current and anticipated efforts to transform the health care landscape through the integration of these principles, and opportunities specific to TBI that such a transformation could seize upon.

Chapter 4 features stakeholder perspectives on using LHS principles to address priority research questions and care needs. The chapter highlights elements including payment models, sociotechnical infrastructure, feedback loops, and outcome comparisons as mechanisms to identify gaps and barriers to effective TBI treatment and to develop strategies to create systems that better meet patient and institutional needs. Chapter 5 offers illustrative examples of current TBI initiatives that employ LHS principles to support care delivery, improve health outcomes, and expand research opportunities. The chapter spotlights advances in TBI interventions, innovative tools, surveillance, and the knowledge base achieved via LHS practices. Chapter 6 examines efforts by federal and state agencies to capture data, conduct surveillance, and support long-term care needs associated with TBI. The chapter underscores the value of interoperability and data standardization in deepening the understanding of TBI, particularly in terms of prevalence, comorbidity, and outcomes data.

Chapter 7 explores the use of LHSs to build and enhance the TBI response capacity of community systems to combat inequitable TBI outcomes within vulnerable populations and geographic locations. Appendix A contains the reference list. See Appendixes B and C for the workshop statement of task and agenda and Appendix D for brief biographies of speakers, moderators, and planning committee members.

2

Lived Experiences

Key Points Highlighted by Individual Speakers[1]

- Navigating health care and health insurance systems to access effective treatment for traumatic brain injury (TBI) requires executive functioning skills that are often compromised by TBI. (Simpson)
- In the current health system, the onus is on the patient to convey information between providers; incentives could serve as a mechanism to encourage collaborative communication between providers. (Simpson)
- TBI specialists could serve as "quarterbacks" for patients, linking them to TBI-focused providers and developing coordinated treatment plans. (Simpson)
- TBI providers should cater to the needs of their patients by implementing practices such as soft lighting and low noise volume in their medical offices, streamlining paperwork processes for medical forms, and using digital appointment reminder systems. (Simpson)

---

[1] This list reflects the rapporteurs' summary of points made by the identified speakers, and the statements have not been endorsed or verified by the National Academies of Sciences, Engineering, and Medicine. They are not intended to reflect a consensus among workshop participants.

- The cost of TBI treatment is prohibitive for many patients; certain treatments are deemed experimental by insurers and therefore not covered by insurance plans. (Simpson)
- Providers should educate and support patients regarding potentially beneficial nonmedical interventions, such as dietary changes, brain exercise, and adaptive tools such as light-filtering contact lenses and noise-canceling headphones. (Simpson)

The first session of the workshop featured a firsthand account of the experiences and consequences of traumatic brain injury (TBI), from its symptoms and their effects on everyday life to barriers to recovery, including the fragmentation of health care and records. Corinne Peek-Asa, vice chancellor for research at University of California, San Diego, moderated the session.

THE EFFECT OF DATA FRAGMENTATION
ON THE EXPERIENCE OF SEEKING AND RECEIVING CARE

Lindsay Simpson, cofounder of the Champion Comeback Foundation, offered a personal account of her efforts to recover from TBI and highlighted changes in the health care system that could better support TBI patients. Although each TBI is unique, there are similarities in symptoms and recovery challenges across the millions of Americans living with these injuries, she said. In 2018, Simpson experienced her eighth documented TBI. Previously able to speak at ease without preparation, she now relies on notes to maintain her train of thought, is unable to memorize lines, and has a lingering speech impediment. In the 2 decades since her first TBI, Simpson has reevaluated her strengths and weaknesses, adapting to areas of deficiency and shifting talents. As her dreams and ambitions have evolved, she has remained determined to continue to improve her functioning and quality of life.

The lack of TBI visibility—both outwardly and on diagnostic imaging—makes the injury and its consequences no less real, she said. Despite people's assurances that she "looks fine," Simpson is always aware of the ways in which her TBIs affect her. For instance, she has no sensation in her right leg, neuropathy on her hands, extreme photo and noise sensitivity, and fatigue; she also experiences double vision because her eyes do not converge properly. Describing her life as "a trail of post-it notes, phone reminders, and routines" required to manage her family, foundation, and consulting business, Simpson stated that regaining basic executive functioning skills has required over 4 years of sessions with a TBI-specific psychologist. "My heart breaks every time my 2-year-old asks me to read him a story, and I can't," she shared.

Simpson's first TBI occurred more than 2 decades ago when she was in 10th grade, resulting in a year's hiatus from sports and significant decreases in her grades and standardized test scores. Common medical advice at the time encouraged people with concussions to stay home in a dark room and avoid exercising the body or brain. She returned to soccer and played at the collegiate level for the University of Maryland. During a game her sophomore year, she experienced her fifth documented TBI during a collision, which ended both her soccer career and her plans to become a cardiothoracic surgeon, as she was no longer able to take classes that required intense memorization. The effects of the TBI required her to change her life goals. She became a sideline reporter for a major league soccer team and vice president of marketing and communications, but shortly before a 2018 broadcast, a 40-pound railing in the newly constructed stadium came loose and struck the side of her head, causing her eighth TBI. In the past 5 years, Simpson has seen over 30 doctors, surgeons, therapists, psychologists, psychiatrists, and other specialists in a quest for relief from pain and other TBI symptoms. She spent much of the first year after the 2018 injury in bed, feeling weak and dazed and experiencing intense migraines. She had two surgeries, received multiple injections, and at times was taking as many as 20 pills each day. Reestablishing typical abilities—such as dressing herself in the morning and driving at night—has required physical, vestibular, speech, occupational, ocular, and cognitive behavioral therapies.

Given the level of intervention required to regain functionality, people contending with TBI symptoms need support navigating the health care system, said Simpson. Scheduling appointments, researching specialists that understand and treat TBI-specific injuries, and navigating health insurance are activities that require healthy executive functioning. To receive the care needed to improve, patients are expected to handle processes made challenging by their symptoms. Simpson highlighted how fragmentation of health care records, the lack of proper exchange of health information, and uncoordinated care among physicians and therapists exacerbate the challenges patients face, noting the trial and error involved in finding a helpful medical team, as not all neurologists specialize in TBI and not all providers understand it. The health system places the onus of conveying information between various doctors and therapists on the patient, she said. However, she often forgot details and became frustrated repeating the same information time and again.

TBI patients need the support of a "quarterback" to effectively navigate health care systems, said Simpson. A quarterback could assist in finding appropriate providers, explaining symptoms in a way doctors understand,

and directing care from a collaborative approach. Simpson found such a quarterback in her primary care physician (PCP), who has been willing to aggregate her test results and quickly fill prescriptions when a specialist is not responding to refill requests. As helpful as this PCP has been in filling care gaps, she does not have specialized TBI knowledge. Simpson emphasized the potential value of TBI specialists serving in this role by developing robust networks of TBI-focused providers and focusing the care team with a cohesive strategy. Outside of a small number of comprehensive TBI centers, she reflected, such quarterbacks do not exist in the current health system. Despite having worked with various case managers, she asserted that none of these professionals effectively bridged health care silos. Case managers tend to have excessive patient loads, little to no clinical experience, and limited networks outside of their disciplines. She found that working with case managers can sometimes increase frustration with the health system rather than alleviate it. While supporting patients, a TBI quarterback could decrease wasteful expenditures in the medical system by shifting from reactive to proactive care, preventing patients from seeing multiple specialists in the search of finding one who truly understands TBI, and avoiding duplicate tests run by multiple providers.

Simpson noted that such support could help patients feel less isolated and adversarial. These feelings are common in a system that often does not take common challenges for patients into consideration. For example, many offices require patients to complete multipage forms in small font in a waiting room with fluorescent lights and a television loudly playing. She has found that some offices do not provide digital or phone appointment reminders despite her requests for such reminders. In the weeks after her TBI, she relied on her husband—whose employer provided the accommodation of working from home to enable him to continue working full-time—to assist her in completing simple tasks such as making coffee, getting dressed, and arriving at appointments. The TBI significantly limited her functioning, yet her neurologist's office expected her to keep up with a paper card to remember the date and time of her visits.

She offered the analogy of an orthopedics office located on the fifth floor of a building without an elevator to describe the lack of consideration some providers give to the TBI patient population. This lack of consideration puts patients on the defensive and could be addressed by using floor lamps in lieu of overhead lighting, offering accommodations for questionnaires, turning off televisions, and investing in a digital appointment reminder system, she suggested. In addition to symptoms, many TBI patients are experiencing great loss—such as loss of identity, friends, athletic career, and/or profession—and they may perceive a lack of accommodation as an indication that providers do not fully understand their needs or that their challenges do not matter.

The cost of health care can be prohibitive for many people with TBI, Simpson emphasized. In her 2 decades contending with TBIs, the most effective treatment she has received was a bilateral suboccipital nerve decompression performed by a neurosurgeon. This procedure significantly reduced her debilitating migraines and caused no discernible side effects. Although this procedure changed her life for the better, insurance denied coverage by declaring it experimental, and she and her husband were responsible for the $40,000 expense out of pocket.

Her medications, injections, therapies, and doctor appointments over the years have totaled to hundreds of thousands of dollars, a sum that most Americans are unable to raise. She believes she could benefit from the collaborative approaches offered in the few comprehensive brain injury clinics in the United States, but most of them are inpatient, they require patients to reside in the area for several months, they carry price tags ranging from $30,000 to $50,000, and they are not covered by her insurance because they are categorized as experimental. Simpson voiced her frustration regarding denial of treatment that could decrease chronic symptoms and the lack of efficient pathways for coverage.

Although she continues to contend with chronic symptoms, the nerve release surgery and several practices have aided her recovery. She noted tremendous improvement in her symptoms when she adopted a low-sugar, high antioxidant, anti-inflammatory diet. Noting that she arrived at this nutrition plan via independent research and initiative, she recommended that TBI patient care plans include nutrition information. To exercise her brain by learning new skills, she challenged herself by pursuing bread baking, furniture refinishing, and gardening. Adaptive tools such as light-filtering contact lenses and noise-canceling headphones have decreased confusion brought on by overstimulation. Before adopting the tools, a trip to the grocery store often became disorienting and unnerving. As with nutrition, she learned about these tools not from doctors but from her own research and networking efforts. The lack of resources for others contending with TBI to discover such information led her and her husband to create the Champion Comeback Foundation. She emphasized that without her dedicated, problem-solving husband, she would not have improved as much as she has. Not all people suffering from TBI symptoms have a strong personal support network, she said, and the health care system should close gaps and adjust practices to better meet their needs.

Although Simpson's experiences are her own, her frustrations are not unique within the TBI community. In preparation for this talk, she explained that she reached out to fellow TBI survivors for input on concerns to emphasize. Danielle, a nurse practitioner who experienced a severe TBI in a 2019 car crash, stated that only those who have suffered a TBI can understand how pervasive its effects are, touching every aspect of life.

She added that practices that have generated the most improvement are often disregarded by allopathic care providers. Jason, a professional soccer player, experienced a series of head injuries until a TBI necessitated his retirement from the sport. He remarked that the U.S. health care system is set up as an authoritative model of dependency in which providers have authority and power. Simpson commented that patients are experts on their bodies in terms of what helps or fails to help; providers should thus encourage and empower patients to pursue any practices that may foster healing. Furthermore, providers should emphasize that the body is always in a state of healing and provide guidance to patients in facilitating that healing. In addition to administering medications, nerve blocks, surgery, and Botox injections, providers can recommend therapies, exercise, nutrition, hydration, supplements, sleep, breath work, meditation, journaling, creative endeavors, and even laughter.

As many as 4 million U.S. athletes will suffer TBI this year, said Simpson. The Champion Comeback Foundation works to connect people contending with a TBI to a network of support and resources, including effective providers in their area.[2] Simpson's husband, Nathan Getty, uses his firsthand experience as a caregiver to fuel his efforts to provide information and support to caregivers. She closed by remarking on the astounding ability of the brain to continually repair and recover, and she called on the expert audience to hold steady in their commitment to addressing the problems she and other TBI patients experience.

DISCUSSION

Caregiver Engagement

Peek-Asa asked about opportunities to engage caregivers in the acute care phase of treatment after TBI and beyond. Simpson remarked that TBI is isolating for both the patient and the caregiver. Life shifted dramatically for her husband when she experienced her eighth TBI. Only 6 weeks into their marriage, Getty was suddenly responsible for helping her with dressing and ensuring she did not leave on the gas stove. Lacking a peer-support network to consult about what to do when one's spouse leaves the stove on for 10 hours or becomes lost at the grocery store, he felt isolated. His work in the foundation is focused on creating such a network for other caregivers in similar situations. She added that support from his employer has been important to her recovery. Understanding that Getty would be better able to be a productive employee if he knew his wife were safe, his employers

---

[2] More information about the Champion Comeback Foundation is available at https://www.championcomeback.org/ (accessed November 10, 2023).

have provided accommodations that allow him to provide needed care while continuing as a full-time employee. Greater awareness of this dynamic could encourage other companies to be similarly accommodating, she suggested.

Health System Data and Collaboration

Peek-Asa asked about features to include or avoid in building medical records and data repositories for TBI. Simpson remarked that while numerous methods of sharing medical notes between providers exist, providers rarely communicate directly with one another about mutual patients. In some cases, a TBI patient may be under the care of a neuropsychologist, a neuropsychiatrist, a TBI neurologist, and a nerve neurologist, all of whom are working within silos and not communicating with one another, aside from sharing notes they may skim during appointments. Acknowledging that building time into providers' schedules for collaborative communication among providers as well as with the patient and/or their caregivers would constitute a substantial change to the current structure, she stated that incentives could be used to spur this needed change. Data systems that require patients to complete increasing amounts of paperwork—particularly in cases where patients are asked to repeatedly fill out the same information—would be ill informed. She added that it can be emotionally taxing for a patient to share current challenges while a provider is typing the entire time. Although notes are needed, time spent typing can undermine connecting with the patient.

Bruce Evans, immediate past president of the National Association of Emergency Medical Technicians, commented that the type of practices used by tumor boards—a convention of providers that discusses treatment plans for patients with cancerous tumors—could serve as a model for interdisciplinary conversations between providers. James Kelly, professor of neurology at the University of Colorado School of Medicine, remarked on the need to enable the workforce pipeline required for providing comprehensive, collaborative TBI care. David Okonkwo, professor of neurological surgery and director of the Neurotrauma Clinical Trials Center at the University of Pittsburgh, commented that the National Academies' Forum on Traumatic Brain Injury was born from the challenge of garnering a sufficient workforce to address the issues Simpson raised by shifting public health, military health, and the larger health care system, noting that forum members are working to deliver more objective diagnostic approaches to TBI and to scale multidisciplinary TBI clinic models. He highlighted the overarching need for care systems to learn from existing models of excellence in TBI care, identify how such models could be duplicated and scaled, and establish frameworks that support system learning, a topic of this workshop, all while staying rooted in the needs of each TBI patient. This critical effort, he suggested, will improve care for the next person to experience TBI.

Medical Disregard of Symptoms

Ramon Diaz-Arrastia, director of the Traumatic Brain Injury Clinical Research Center at the University of Pennsylvania, noted the limited availability of diagnostic tools for many TBIs and asked whether Simpson ever felt that medical professionals discounted her experience as a psychiatric issue. She replied that her life would be substantially different if diagnostic tools could confirm her diagnosis, relieving her of the burden of continually trying to prove to doctors, family, and friends that her symptoms are real. Recounting a doctor who told her she was depressed because she cried in the office, she stated that crying spells are caused by dysregulation of her emotions and are accompanied by outbursts of yelling. "I'm not depressed; I'm scared," Simpson remarked, sharing that in the midst of great loss she has had to face the difficulty of having doctors tell her that they do not know what is wrong with her or providing a rationale for her symptoms that make no sense, such as a doctor who told her the absence of sensation in her leg was attributable to wearing a heavy tool belt despite the fact that she has never worn a tool belt. The need to prove her symptoms are real is only strengthened when medical offices appear to ignore common TBI symptoms by featuring bright lights and loud televisions in their waiting rooms.

Emergency Medical Services

Evans asked whether emergency medical services (EMS) attended to Simpson after any of her TBIs and her experience of how such prehospital services connected to hospital care and data systems, to inform integration and learning. Given the bright lights, crowded waiting rooms, and collection of sounds common in emergency departments (EDs), Simpson replied that she stubbornly avoids visits to the ED if at all possible. Although she was treated in the ED after some of her TBIs, her most recent and severe TBI was treated by EMS personnel on site at the stadium. After she refused an ED visit, the team doctor treated her and provided clearance for her to seek treatment with him the following day in lieu of going to the ED.

Brain Function and Diet

Noting Simpson's comments that she needed to take initiative to identify practices that supported her brain wellness, Beth McQuiston, neurologist, dietitian, and medical director of diagnostics at Abbott Laboratories, remarked on the role of nutrition, healthy living, and alternative practices in optimizing brain function. The lipid membranes of the brain are composed of dietary components, including polyphenols and antioxidants. Thus, diet can have a notable effect on brain function. In recommending brain-healthy diets, she said, providers can empower and encourage patients in their healing.

3

The Learning Health System

Key Points Highlighted by Individual Speakers[1]

- A learning health system (LHS) aligns science, informatics, incentives, and culture for continuous improvement, innovation, and equity. (McGinnis)
- A quality health system is patient engaged, safe, effective, equitable, efficient, accessible, transparent, measurable, secure, and adaptive. (McGinnis)
- Networks formed within the National Academy of Medicine Leadership Consortium are developing strategies to scale LHS principles and activities related to culture, informatics, incentives, and science. (McGinnis)

The second session of the workshop featured an overview of the learning health system (LHS) concept and efforts to shift health systems toward such a model. Odette Harris, professor of neurosurgery at Stanford University and deputy chief of staff for rehabilitation at the Veterans Affairs Palo Alto Health Care System, moderated the session.

---

[1] This list reflects the rapporteurs' summary of points made by the identified speakers, and the statements have not been endorsed or verified by the National Academies of Sciences, Engineering, and Medicine. They are not intended to reflect a consensus among workshop participants.

LEARNING HEALTH CARE SYSTEMS

J. Michael McGinnis, Leonard D. Schaefer Executive Officer of the National Academy of Medicine (NAM), discussed the development of the LHS definition and its core principles, as well as current efforts to expand and scale this concept. He remarked on the tremendous opportunity to accelerate progress in applying the LHS approach to traumatic brain injuries (TBI). Given the $4 trillion spent annually on health care in the United States, the resources and the technology required to develop systems that learn and advance from every patient experience are available, he said, provided the will to dedicate resources to this endeavor is mustered.

Strategy for Creating Learning Health Care Systems

McGinnis explained that the strategy for building LHSs was born from two reports from the Institute of Medicine (IOM) (2000, 2001). These reports—which emphasized a focus on quality and safety—established the core principles that health care should be patient centered, safe, effective, equitable, efficient, and timely. As a lack of robust effectiveness data for many medical interventions became apparent, the issue of effectiveness emerged as a particular concern. Responding to a charge from the insurance and manufacturing sectors, IOM established the Roundtable on Evidence-Based Medicine in 2005. This group soon identified an absence of evidence for many common medical practices. Given the impracticality of conducting 5-year, $100 million randomized controlled trials (RCTs) to fill each data gap, the roundtable looked to new research methodologies and technologies to accelerate the process for developing a continuous LHS. A 2006 workshop and subsequent activities advanced an understanding of the LHS concept, with McGinnis described as

> a health system in which science, informatics, incentives, and culture are aligned for continuous improvement, innovation, and equity—with best practices and discoveries seamlessly embedded in the delivery process, individuals and families as active participants in all elements, and new knowledge generated as an integral byproduct of the delivery experience.

Furthermore, he noted that acceleration toward such a movement would require the involvement of manufacturers, insurers, health professionals, digital infrastructure stewards, and patients and families.

Working toward that end, the roundtable formed a vision of developing the defined LHS, McGinnis said. The group created a series of action collaboratives based on the four elements featured in the LHS definition: evidence mobilization (science), digital health (informatics), incentives and systems, and inclusion and equity (culture). These action collaboratives developed agendas identifying key pressure points to use in their respective arenas to achieve an LHS. The transformation targets across collaboratives include digital infrastructure, health and social data, effectiveness research, technical innovation, financial incentives, person and family engagement, community activation, and the decision culture. In exploring these various elements, the collaboratives produced over 30 publications in the Learning Health System series.[2]

Each action collaborative established goals within four strategic action domains—digital, evidence, economics, and sociocultural:

- Digital strategic action goals focus on developing a virtual health data trust in which data are interoperable, accessible, and protected.
- Evidence goals center on increasing real world learning capacity, including RCTs in some—but not all—cases. McGinnis emphasized the importance of ensuring that expensive, time-consuming RCTs remain relevant when they reach completion, not having become outdated during the years the process entails.
- Economic action goals target alignment of resources with health outcomes and a shift from fee-for-service as the major driver to payment for outcomes that matter most to individuals and to communities.
- Sociocultural goals focus on full and equitable health engagement.

Applying Core Principles to Practice

After much exploration of these complex issues, several action collaborative initiatives are poised to move forward, McGinnis said. The spread and scale of core principles is most imminent. As shown in Figure 3-1, the core principles of a quality health system originally identified in the IOM reports have been expanded. Initial *patient centered* terminology shifted to *engaged* to reflect active patient participation in a system fundamentally oriented to a partnership between patients, families, and the clinical enterprise. *Timely* has been replaced by *accessible* to encapsulate both timing and access in the ready availability of services. And four additional principles have been added: *transparent, accountable, secure, and adaptive.* A *transparent* system provides clear information related to the nature, use, costs, and results of services. *Accountable* refers to the reliable assessment of consequential activities and outcomes. McGinnis also emphasized that a system focused on outcomes does not attempt to measure every step of a

---

[2] See the Learning Health System series at https://nam.edu/programs/value-science-driven-health-care/learning-health-system-series/ (accessed February 5, 2024).

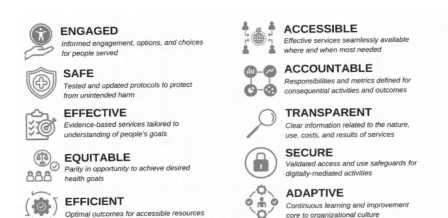

ENGAGED
Informed engagement, options, and choices for people served

SAFE
Tested and updated protocols to protect from unintended harm

EFFECTIVE
Evidence-based services tailored to understanding of people's goals

EQUITABLE
Parity in opportunity to achieve desired health goals

EFFICIENT
Optimal outcomes for accessible resources

ACCESSIBLE
Effective services seamlessly available where and when most needed

ACCOUNTABLE
Responsibilities and metrics defined for consequential activities and outcomes

TRANSPARENT
Clear information related to the nature, use, costs, and results of services

SECURE
Validated access and use safeguards for digitally-mediated activities

ADAPTIVE
Continuous learning and improvement core to organizational culture

FIGURE 3-1 Core principles of a learning health system.
SOURCE: Presented by Michael McGinnis, October 12, 2023. National Academy of Medicine Leadership Consortium: Collaboration for a Learning Health System (available at https://nam.edu/lhs-core-principles).

process, but rather measures what matters most for the individual, the care delivery system, and the community. A *secure* system offers validated access and uses safeguards for digitally mediated activities. An *adaptive* system has an organizational culture with continuous learning and improvement at its core.

The roundtable is currently partnering with the American Hospital Association, the American Medical Association, state medical boards, and a broad range of participants to ensure that institutions and providers nationwide are stewards in creating learning health organizations, said McGinnis. This effort will also engage the National Institutes of Health, the Centers for Disease Control and Prevention, the Health Resources and Services Administration, and major organizations in the NAM Leadership Consortium. Given the fragmented nature of the U.S. health care system, the establishment of common commitments provides reference points for organizations working to improve the ways in which they engage with patients, he stated. The action collaboratives are building a series of networks focused on culture, informatics, incentives, and science to advance strategies to scale LHS principles and activities. As this effort progresses, these networks will also provide a mechanism for gathering information. He emphasized that the professionals working to develop and spread new LHS initiatives are pioneers and are valuable in helping to identify opportunities.

The collaboratives have developed starter application templates describing how the core principles apply within the arenas of culture, informatics, incentives, and science, McGinnis explained. He provided examples of how each of the 10 core principles applies to the areas of digital health and evidence mobilization (see Box 3-1). McGinnis emphasized that organizations should adapt and expand these starter applications to their circumstances. In working toward the core principles across the arenas of evidence, informatics, incentives, and culture, organizations can establish LHSs. Furthermore, organizations can consider how these applications apply across sites including the clinic, home, businesses, and communities.

BOX 3-1
Applying Learning Health System Principles in Two Areas

Digital Health

- Engaged: Digital health records reflect engagement when discretion on control and use of personal data resides with the individual or their designee.
- Safe: Safety involves data stewardship protocols that safeguard against use resulting in harm.
- Effective: Digital health records collect and maintain data according to validated stewardship protocols.
- Equitable: Data systems are designed to identify and counter bias or disparities.
- Efficient: Data systems acquire only those service licenses that enhance health system interoperability.
- Accessible: Records feature data that are available at the times, locations, and on devices most proximate to decisions.
- Measurable: Systems continuously monitor digital health performance for accuracy and interoperability.
- Transparent: Transparency is achieved by making the sources and uses of personal data clearly evident.
- Secure: Systems establish data sharing protocols that are transparent and are considered secure by users.
- Adaptive: Adaptability is achieved when data strategies are regularly calibrated to ensure continuity, currency, utility, and security.

Evidence Mobilization

- Engaged: Mobilization occurs when individuals, circumstances, and personal goals shape health and health care.
- Safe: Safety is fostered by health services and research that contain safeguards against unintended harm.
- Effective: Health services both reflect and enhance the evidence base.
- Equitable: Equity involves developing and applying evidence with care and standards to eliminate bias.
- Efficient: Evidence mobilization develops and applies evidence using resource-optimization strategies.

continued

BOX 3-1 Continued

- Accessible: Accessible evidence refers to the availability of best evidence at the point of choice to guide health services delivery.
- Measurable: A measurable system digitally records and assesses health services for continuous learning.
- Transparent: Evidence is open and accountable as to source strength and applicability.
- Secure: Security involves services and results that are tracked, reported, and stored with validated safeguards.
- Adaptive: An adaptive system features evidence, algorithms, and service protocols that reflect the evolving knowledge base.

SOURCE: Presented by Michael McGinnis, October 12, 2023.

McGinnis closed with the example of applying the learning health system approach to an assessment of the impact of the COVID-19 pandemic across the health system, which identified the need for a commission to explore the challenges that system fragmentation, perverse or misaligned incentives, and inequities posed to the pandemic responses (NAM, 2023). To address this need, NAM has established the National Commission on Investment Imperatives for a Healthy Nation to integrate lessons learned and advance alignment across sectors via five work streams: individual and community health goals, inclusive and equitable systems, digital and data architecture, funding and accountability, and private equity health investments.

DISCUSSION

Principle Prioritization

Kathy Lee, senior health policy analyst at the Office of the Deputy Assistant Secretary of Defense for Health Readiness Policy and Oversight, asked about core principles to prioritize during the initial stages of creating a learning health care system. McGinnis replied that the core principles can serve as a checklist for health organizations to use in reviewing their performance within each dimension. The results of such a review may lead different organizations to varied emphases. An initial priority for a TBI system should be engaging patients, families, and communities, he suggested, noting that a financial reimbursement system for medical care will not precede grassroots demand and political will for this care. Lee asked about the size and scope desired in a learning health care system. McGinnis clarified that the entire system of factors that impinge on health status are involved, including public health, social services, organizations, and constituent groups.

Cross-Sector Collaboration

Christina Master, pediatrician and sports medicine specialist at Children's Hospital of Philadelphia, noted the critical role of electronic health records and health information systems in caring for children with mild TBI. She asked about strategies for engaging partners from industry and academia, given that goals may differ and, in some cases, competitive interests may be at play. McGinnis emphasized the value of discussing common commitments with partners across sectors, specifically and transparently voicing the implications of moving forward. The development of generative artificial intelligence (AI) and large language models holds potential to transform the way business is conducted and how patients and families are engaged in the learning enterprise, he said.

Measuring and Replicating Excellence

Ramon Diaz-Arrastia, director of the Traumatic Brain Injury Clinical Research Center at the University of Pennsylvania, remarked that the fragmented U.S. health system presents challenges, but it also enables innovation and excellence to emerge organically. Given that a top-down system is unlikely to function well over the long term, he asked how best to identify centers of excellence and disseminate their models. McGinnis replied that while a top-down system is unlikely to take root, a more integrated system delivering evidence-based interventions is possible. Such a system should operate with a governance structure that generates transparency regarding the results of interventions and common approaches to health care delivery, he said, and an inherent challenge in this process is the need to narrow down measurement strategies to a relatively small number. For instance, IOM issued a report that examined 2,000 measures required by Medicare, Medicaid, and other insurance systems, then identified key clusters among those measures and described how AI and machine learning could be used to ease data collection and assessment (IOM, 2015). Regarding centers of excellence, McGinnis noted that roundtable action collaboratives have identified best practices related to informatics, evidence, culture, and incentives and will feature these in an upcoming annual report.

Health Outcomes and Spending

The session moderator Harris commented that health system incentives can be at odds with a patient-engagement model; she asked how to address this pervasive barrier. McGinnis emphasized that an understanding of what patients and families need in order to meet their goals must drive the process, and incentives then must be structured accordingly. Incentives for outcomes will only be built into systems with full partnership and advocacy from the patient and family community. Currently, he said, the U.S. health care system spends $4 trillion annually, and a quarter of this expense is waste (CMS, 2023; Shrank et al., 2019). This waste is reflected in the country's rank of 35th worldwide in performance (in terms of outcomes) despite outspending all other countries. Furthermore, the current incentive system has enabled intractable inequities. He emphasized that political will is needed to change the incentive system and, to this end, experts should partner with patients and families to identify the consequences of this system in a cohesive and compelling manner.

4

Use of Learning Health Care Systems to Improve Care for Traumatic Brain Injury

---

Key Points Highlighted by Individual Speakers[1]

- Payment models can be used as mechanisms to foster positive patient outcomes by increasing care affordability, coordination, and access. (Davidson)
- Sociotechnical infrastructure enables each clinical department or unit to function as a learning health system (LHS), which can then aggregate to a collective LHS at the larger organizational level. (Lomotan)
- Feedback loops foster the development of knowledge and situational awareness within a health system. Building feedback loops, capturing higher-quality data, and conducting randomized trials are LHS strategies appropriate for improving traumatic brain injury (TBI) care. (Horwitz)
- The Department of Veterans Affairs strives to offer integrated, individualized, and interdisciplinary delivery of quality, long-term TBI care that maximizes patient outcomes. Data collection and analysis of outcome comparisons inform the developing LHS. (Scholten)

---

[1] This list reflects the rapporteurs' summary of points made by the identified speakers, and the statements have not been endorsed or verified by the National Academies of Sciences, Engineering, and Medicine. They are not intended to reflect a consensus among workshop participants.

- The Center for Medicare and Medicaid Innovation is building feedback loops with providers, patients, and patient organizations to better understand patient needs and establish incentives to encourage practices that meet those needs. (Davidson)
- Organizations should strive to collect findable, accessible, interoperable, reusable, and computable data that enable learning transfer. (Lomotan)
- Approaches that can help rural or less well-resourced systems develop and participate in learning health systems include providing financial or payment system incentives, incorporating virtual care options, and making use of strategies such as simple randomization to test and learn from different practices. (Davidson, Horwitz, Lomotan, Scholten)

The third session of the workshop featured stakeholder perspectives on how learning health systems (LHSs) can address unmet priorities that apply to traumatic brain injury (TBI). The session discussed the Centers for Medicare and Medicaid Services (CMS) Innovation Center's role in testing, learning, and scaling approaches for more effective care delivery and payment; the digital and analytic infrastructure needed to develop and maintain LHSs, examples of operationalizing LHS principles at New York University (NYU) Langone Health, and how the Department of Veterans Affairs models the concept of an LHS for veterans with TBI. Participants explored the use of such systems to identify gaps, barriers, and strategies to effectively address institutional needs, including how their organizations use data and innovation to improve health care delivery. David Goldstein, senior advisor at the Department of Health and Human Services, moderated the session.

PERSPECTIVES PANEL

Center for Medicare and Medicaid Innovation

Kathryn Davidson, director of the learning and diffusion group at the Center for Medicare and Medicaid Innovation (CMMI), described the development of payment models to support patient outcomes. A licensed clinical social worker, she began her career overseeing randomized clinical trials in community settings. At this intersection of behavioral health, social services, and primary care, she witnessed the profound effect of loss of grant funding on outcomes. Her work at CMMI enables her to direct her implementation science focus on the development of payment models that foster positive patient outcomes and feature flexibilities that engage patients and caregivers. Born from the 2010 Affordable Care Act, CMMI tests new payment models that aim to reduce health care costs and increase quality. The organization works to improve patient outcomes by narrowing quality measures and by identifying incentives and flexibilities that promote innovation at the point of care delivery. Noting the high threshold of simultaneously reducing cost and improving quality, she reported that CMMI has tested approximately 50 models, but only 4 have been scaled to date. Innovation in care delivery is not limited to tested models, and CMMI's learning and diffusion group and evaluation teams work to examine, understand, and enable innovative practices that benefit patients. As innovators develop practices that increase the patient experience of affordability, coordination, and access, CMMI considers the payment models needed to encourage these practices.

Agency for Healthcare Research and Quality

Edwin Lomotan, senior advisor for clinical informatics in the Center for Evidence and Practice Improvement at the Agency for Healthcare Research and Quality (AHRQ), discussed his organization's role in providing tools, resources, and funding to support the development of LHSs. The agency's mission is to produce evidence to improve the safety, quality, accessibility, equity, and affordability of health care, as well as ensuring the use of evidence in the field. For example, the AHRQ Evidence-Based Practice Center program produced a series of evidence reports on LHSs featuring topics such as engaging patients, families, and caregivers and addressing diagnostic errors. The agency's activities to support patient-centered outcomes research include training LHS researchers. The program that Lomotan leads focuses on advancing patient-centered clinical decision support, which is relevant to LHSs and incorporating perspectives from patients, families, and caregivers. In addition, he is currently among a group convened by the University of Michigan and AcademyHealth that is developing an LHS maturity model that identifies the stages of a health care system transitioning to becoming an LHS. Sociotechnical infrastructure provides the personnel, processes, and technologies needed to create a system in which each unit of a health system—such as a TBI care center—functions as a small-scale LHS. These units can then collectively operate as an LHS at the organizational level, which incorporates and expands learnings across the organization and creates a whole greater than the sums of its parts.

New York University Langone Health

Leora Horwitz, director of the Center for Healthcare Innovation and Delivery Science at NYU Langone Health, explored strategies to shift health systems toward becoming LHSs. The complexity of health care systems poses challenges to understanding how all parts operate. Feedback loops are a mechanism for developing knowledge and situational awareness about the health system. An effort to promote flu shots exemplifies this dynamic. Each September, NYU Langone Health activates an electronic alert instructing nurses to administer flu shots to patients. Several years ago, Horwitz and colleagues realized that the flu shot alert was initiated 22 times per patient per day, and was ignored 99.5 percent of the time, even though it resulted in 90 percent of eligible patients receiving the vaccination prior to discharge. After soliciting feedback from nurses, the team made several changes to the alert, but this effort only decreased the alerts by one per patient per day. A link added to the alert enabled recipients to provide comments, resulting in large quantities of varied feedback. This feedback loop revealed that the alert was issued within operating rooms (ORs), postanesthesia care units, endoscopy suites, and other locations where flu shots are not administered. The team then recognized that the information technology (IT) department set the alert to initiate each time a health professional updated the patient flow sheet. Although the flow sheet is updated about four to six times a day in many parts of the hospital, update rates within the OR are sometimes as frequent as once per minute. Despite the long-standing frustration that incessant flu shot alerts caused OR nurses, a mechanism for them to communicate this to IT was lacking. Once Horwitz's team identified the issue, flu vaccine alerts were limited to only appropriate units within the hospital, resulting in a rate of five alerts per patient per day. She highlighted that establishing mechanisms to solicit patient feedback is a primary strategy in creating an LHS. For example, feedback loops could inform staff in medical offices that the television volume and lighting brightness are causing discomfort for their TBI patients.

Generation of higher-quality data is a secondary strategy to employ in shifting systems toward becoming LHSs, said Horwitz. Although data are plentiful in health systems, the ability to collect and convert meaningful data into knowledge is often limited. Health systems typically gather data points rather than use a structured approach that captures synthesis, judgment, experience, trajectory, and thought processes. She offered the example of a project several years ago aimed at optimizing testing in the emergency department (ED) for pulmonary emboli (PE) blood clots in the lungs. These clots can be catastrophic, yet they are easy to miss. Testing involves a computed tomography (CT) scan with radiation and contrast; therefore, it is not feasible or advisable to administer to all patients in the ED. Horwitz's team built an automatic PE risk score calculation into the software system. When a physician ordered a CT scan for a person with a low PE risk score, the system issued an alert that suggested a preliminary D-dimer test before proceeding with the CT scan. Recognizing that these alerts were often ignored, the team solicited feedback from ED doctors about the PE risk scoring calculation. Several physicians noted that because of NYU's proximity to John F. Kennedy International Airport, the hospital frequently treats patients who have traveled on long overseas flights and have blood clots in their legs; however, the scoring system does not account for the PE risk that travel poses. Some doctors cited patients with prominent family histories of blood clots. Others explained they have honed their intuition over decades of experience.

To gather more data, Horwitz's team added a system prompt that asked doctors to input their reason for overriding the low PE risk alert, such as recent travel, a hypercoagulable state, or high clinical suspicion. After several months of data collection, analysis revealed that CT scans ordered for patients because of recent travel rarely found blood clots. However, when doctors noted clinical suspicion of PE for patients with a low automatic risk calculation, the rate of PE was much higher. The center used this knowledge in reeducating doctors regarding their intuition, encouraging them to trust their judgment in some cases and advising them against overweighing certain factors that did not significantly increase the risk for PE. Horwitz stated that a TBI LHS could solicit feedback from providers about whether they suspect a patient has a TBI, the predicted trajectory, and treatments they predict as likely to be effective. A feedback loop could collect and analyze such data to inform TBI care.

The ability to generate readily and rigorously evaluable data is not reliant on receiving large grants, said Horwitz, noting that her team at NYU Langone Health has conducted approximately 30 randomized trials in the absence of funding from the National Institutes of Health. One such trial arose in response to the substantial decline in pediatric vaccination rates during the COVID-19 pandemic. Her team solicited feedback from parents of pediatric patients in order to target text message reminders. Parents offered reasons for delayed vaccination that included fear of contracting COVID-19 while in the clinic, the time commitment required to attend appointments, and a lack of understanding the rationale for vaccination. The team created several reminder messages with varied content and randomized delivery of the text messages to parents. None of the messages resulted in significant vaccination increases compared to the control group not receiving reminders.

Again reaching out for feedback, the team called parents to ask whether they had received the text messages and why they had not acted on them. Most of the parents indicated the lack of follow through was attributable to receiving the reminders while they were at work or when the clinic was closed, rendering them unable to call and make the appointment. The team conducted an additional randomized trial in which one group of parents received an initial text message in the evening that included a link to online appointment scheduling and a second message sent 36 hours later at lunch time. The vaccination rate among children with parents in this group tripled in comparison to the control group not receiving a reminder. After randomized trials revealed the role of staggered text reminders in increasing vaccination, the practice was adopted systemwide. The LHS strategies of building feedback loops, capturing higher-quality data, and conducting randomized trials help illustrate opportunities applicable to advancing learning systems for TBI care.

Veterans Affairs Washington, DC, Health Care System

Joel Scholten, executive director of Physical Medicine & Rehabilitation at the Department of Veterans Affairs (VA), described efforts to incorporate integrated interdisciplinary TBI teams into a developing LHS. He noted that although VA features over 100 TBI teams, the VA health care system has over 1,000 points of care delivery; thus, only 10 percent of VA locations include onsite specialized, interdisciplinary TBI care. Drawing from their experience working with both TBI teams and individual veterans, case managers provide highly valued input. Using the electronic health record (EHR), VA created a plan of care templated note that is easily searchable and can be updated as a patient progresses through a treatment plan and transitions to a wellness plan. VA's mission of helping veterans access lifelong care and wellness underlies a shift from episodic care to long-term, quality care that includes inpatient TBI units accredited by the Commission on Accreditation of Rehabilitation Facilities. Extensive VA research efforts—such as long-term implementation studies, partnerships with academic institutions, and collaboration with 16 TBI model systems nationwide—have generated a longitudinal database. Outcome comparisons from these data foster an understanding of the unique health care needs veterans experience following TBI.

Scholten noted a VA caregiver program that provides stipends to reimburse some of the time caregivers dedicate to care. Other VA benefits include home modification, vehicle adaptation, and housing support for homeless veterans. Implementing a whole health model of care, VA is working to shift from a focus on what is the matter with a veteran to what matters to the veteran. This priority seeks to offer integrated, individualized care delivery that maximizes patient engagement and treatment outcomes for veterans.

DISCUSSION

Data Strategies to Develop Learning Health Systems

Goldstein asked how organizations can move an LHS forward strategically and innovatively while integrating considerations such as program evaluation and stakeholder engagement. Davidson noted CMMI efforts to foster patient-centered and value-based care in the context of the large

Centers for Medicare and Medicaid Services (CMS) system, and that these strategies align well with LHS core principles. For example, efforts often seek to create flexibility, use data-driven decision making, center patients, and make use of cohesive payment models to defragment care delivery and improve outcomes. Lessons from such models can inform other organizations' LHS efforts.

Davidson noted challenges in making vast quantities of CMS data usable in order to identify trends in health care. For example, the Medicare skilled nursing facility 3-day inpatient hospital stay waiver was coded with different names in various models. The learning and diffusion group has been systematically identifying such data entry issues to generate consistency and simplify data collection and analysis. Using data from claims, quality measures, learning systems, and evaluations, the group draws conclusions that inform future model development.

Partnering with external stakeholders, CMS capitalizes on its ability to use payment models for point-of-care innovation while learning from care delivery experts about practices that improve patient outcomes. To that end, CMMI is building feedback loops with providers, patients, and patient organizations to better understand what patients need and, in turn, establish incentives to shift practice toward meeting those needs. Thereby, CMMI creates an LHS internally while reinforcing LHS processes externally through partnerships with model participants.

Goldstein asked about data infrastructure innovations that a care system can adopt early in the process of becoming an LHS. Lomotan noted the relevance of a maturity model in considering an organization's starting point from which to compare and track improvement, and stated that data infrastructure strategies will vary between care systems. Data should capture unmet patient needs and practices that are working, he said. Furthermore, organizations should strive to collect data that are findable, accessible, interoperable, reusable, and computable. Various mechanisms for collecting such data include decision logs, use spreadsheets, and systems based on artificial intelligence (AI). With a focus on applying what has been learned across settings and contexts, AHRQ works to analyze data from multiple agencies and has recently developed an application programming interface that indexes repositories and creates interoperable data points that can be used repeatedly for a variety of purposes.

Data and Continuous Improvement

Regarding the creation of a learning system that incorporates up-to-date evidence and establishes a culture of continuous quality improvement, Horwitz emphasized the importance of collaboration with departments and disciplines within a health system when determining areas of evidence-based care in need of support. Rather than dictating changes, she and her team ask providers about pain points patients are experiencing, practices that seem to work but are lacking data, and facets of the program that may not be working well. Next, they collaborate in devising a mechanism to test the practice. She noted that the majority of the time, data on untested practices do not reflect the benefit that providers ascribe to them. These cases are viewed as opportunities for iteration and improvement. For example, the team spent 6 years tweaking the flu vaccine computer alert to achieve a rate of less than one alert per patient per day. The learning process requires time and experimentation, she emphasized, and once a better method is identified, NYU Langone Health generalizes it to routine practice across appropriate departments.

Competing priorities are inherent in a system as large as VA, and data can serve as leverage for assets and resources, said Scholten. In an effort to prioritize TBI needs within the entire VA health system, he works to integrate TBI with other agency-wide priorities. Narratives of individual veterans living with TBI highlight the role of quality care in improving outcomes. TBI teams communicate these stories to the community clinics where many veterans receive treatment. Given the 1,000 points of care delivery within the VA system, medical records can span numerous care locations. VA will soon introduce a new EHR system, and integration of all existing medical records could require a 10-year time frame. Meanwhile, investment in data and programming requests for the existing EHR will be limited. Furthermore, 75 percent of post-9/11 veterans with TBI also have post-traumatic stress disorder and receive care from mental health partners. This holistic model of care increases the complexity of integrating all medical records.

Comprehensive data enable dashboard metrics that aid in identifying frequency of quality-of-care outliers and can be used in improving the practice of individual providers. Over time, the use of data shifts the culture toward evidence-based care, he said. Proactive VA case management uses data to annually identify TBI patients with chronic disability; case managers then follow up with veterans and update wellness plans accordingly. After 2 years of establishing this process, the percentage of veterans with TBI that receive annual, in-person visits with health providers has increased from 20 percent to 50 percent. Goldstein remarked on the interplay of care delivery, organizational structure, data, and technology. As a result, he reflected, consideration should be given to the timing of engaging stakeholders in public and private partnerships to promote transparency while avoiding overburdening the process.

Supporting LHS Efforts Within a Care System

Joseph Giacino, director of rehabilitation neuropsychology at Spaulding Rehabilitation Hospital and professor of physical medicine and rehabilitation at Harvard Medical School, asked about the operational structure of NYU Langone Health's evidence-to-practice feedback cycle. Horwitz replied that the Center for Healthcare Innovation and Delivery Science employs a project manager, two research associates, and two data analysts. She and a senior-level statistician dedicate part of their time to the center. One data analyst is focused on moving data into the EHR, which uses Epic software. Epic features a core function that enables randomization of electronic health alert recipients; thus, other health systems using Epic could conduct experiments similar to the work carried out at NYU with assistance from their IT departments. She emphasized the value of NYU Langone Health's IT collaboration in enabling an iterative process of trial and error. This collaboration is ensured by the chief information officer's commitment to creating an information system that meets the needs of both patients and providers. While grants enable some center activities, NYU Langone Health has funded the core operations of the center for 10 years. Horwitz meets with the executive team on a quarterly basis to ensure that the center's activities are aligned with institutional priorities, further building organizational alignment and support for LHS efforts.

Engaging Health Systems in LHS Efforts

Corinne Peek-Asa, vice chancellor for research at the University of California, San Diego, asked about mechanisms such as incentives to translate knowledge gained across systems, including those in rural areas, and support the ability of less well-resourced systems to implement LHS practices. Scholten replied that VA uses virtual care in helping address inequity in the geographical availability of TBI care centers and that the federal nature of VA enables nationwide use of virtual care, regardless of state boundaries. Davidson noted that CMMI recently analyzed penetration of value-based care to identify types of providers and geographical areas that these models have not yet reached. To address identified gaps and bolster primary care, CMMI is testing models that feature upfront infrastructure, streamlined models and simplified incentives to support more widespread participation in value-based care in alignment with LHS goals. She noted the Making Care Primary model and States Advancing All-Payer Health Equity Approaches and Development (AHEAD) model, aimed at fostering coordinated, high-quality, and cost efficient care across primary and specialty disciples to improve health outcomes.

Lomotan echoed the importance of addressing health inequities in the design stage of an LHS, which needs to incorporate feedback from patients and families in order to build patient-engaged systems that address barriers to care. He emphasized that too often, patient input is not solicited until the end stages of system design.

Horwitz commented that although advanced EHR randomization and AI models can be used to analyze and learn from system data, NYU also uses simple strategies to align practice with LHS principles, and that these strategies can be employed by many types of care systems. For example, a project conducted with a call center alternated between two scripts on a weekly basis and filtered call lists according to medical record numbers being odd or even. These simple methods are not formal randomized trials but can be used to test different options in a wide range of settings with limited research budgets, including rural care settings. She added that NYU Langone Health has a toolkit available on its website to assist with this process.[2]

---

[2] See https://med.nyu.edu/centers-programs/healthcare-innovation-delivery-science/sites/default/files/chids-toolkit.pdf (accessed January 3, 2024).

5

Examples of Learning Health Care Systems in Traumatic Brain Injury

---

Key Points Highlighted by Individual Speakers[1]

- Comparing Treatment Approaches to Promote Inpatient Rehabilitation Effectiveness for Traumatic Brain Injury (CARE4TBI) is a therapist-driven effort to identify effective rehabilitation approaches through data analysis of clinical practice. (Bogner)
- CARE4TBI engaged clinicians in creating standardized data elements for documenting clinical care in the electronic health record that aligned with the priorities of rehabilitation services providers, while providing a format that is amenable to data extraction and analysis. (Bogner)
- A learning health system (LHS) should enable exploration of highly specific questions relevant to patients with traumatic brain injury (TBI). (Giacino)
- The Transforming Research and Clinical Knowledge in TBI study has led to advances in TBI assessment tools such as the Glasgow Outcome Scale-Extended, OsiriX common data elements software for evaluating MRI scans, and TBI blood biomarker rapid testing. (Giacino)

---

[1] This list reflects the rapporteurs' summary of points made by the identified speakers, and the statements have not been endorsed or verified by the National Academies of Sciences, Engineering, and Medicine. They are not intended to reflect a consensus among workshop participants.

- The Department of Defense TBI Center of Excellence has conducted surveillance and data analysis projects to identify military occupational specialties at higher risk for TBI and the prevalence of various comorbidities in the months before and after TBI. (Stout)
- Feedback loops enable systems to better meet the needs of patients and providers and should be implemented early in system design. (Giacino, Stout)
- LHS challenges include medical documentation that is not formatted to allow for outcome and program evaluation, as well as databases that lack interoperability and thus limit data aggregation. (Bogner, Evans, Stout)
- Payment models that support the implementation of identified effective practices are needed to enable provision of TBI care that leads to best outcomes. (Giacino, Harris, Manley)
- Refining how the severity of TBI is classified is a critical step to improving care and outcomes. Also critical are the consideration of factors affecting outcome beyond biology at the time of injury, such as social and environmental factors. (Bogner, Manley)

The fifth session of the workshop featured three traumatic brain injury (TBI) initiatives that are developing learning health systems (LHS) in an effort to improve TBI research, clinical practice, and clinical operations. Session examples highlighted how Comparing Treatment Approaches to Promote Inpatient Rehabilitation Effectiveness for TBI (CARE4TBI) and TRACK-TBI networks advance research on acute injury and longer-term recovery from TBI and seek to connect this knowledge to improved patient outcomes, while analyses of the Department of Defense's TBI surveillance dataset provide insights to inform programs and policies for service members. Nsini Umoh, program director in the National Institute of Neurological Disorders and Stroke (NINDS) Division of Neuroscience repair and plasticity cluster, moderated the session.

CARE4TBI: COMPARING TREATMENT APPROACHES TO PROMOTE INPATIENT REHABILITATION EFFECTIVENESS FOR TRAUMATIC BRAIN INJURY

Jennifer Bogner, professor and Bert C. Wiley, M.D., Endowed Chair in the Department of Physical Medicine and Rehabilitation at the Ohio State University (OSU) Medical Center, provided an overview of CARE4TBI, which is a comprehensive investigation of real-life rehabilitation approaches to identify interventions that are effective at various points in the recovery process.[2] Interventions are based on lessons learned from more than a decade of preliminary studies, the infrastructure of the National Institute on Disability, Independent Living, and Rehabilitation Research (NIDILRR) TBI Model Systems program, and stakeholder engagement.[3] The CARE4TBI study aims to develop standardized data elements within electronic health records (EHRs) across sites to enable data extraction for research purposes and clinical operations. The study has just begun its next phase, which uses causal inference methods to compare the effectiveness of various rehabilitation approaches. She noted that although CARE4TBI is creating an LHS foundation, the process of becoming a fully functioning LHS is still underway.

Drawing from practice-based data on TBI care, existing projects serve as key components for CARE4TBI, Bogner explained. A 1998 consensus conference on TBI held by the National Institutes of Health concluded that inpatient rehabilitation is effective, though not fully understood, and called for additional research to identify the interventions and other factors responsible for desired outcomes (NIH Panel, 1999). The TBI Practice-Based Evidence study in 10 North American sites provided insight on rehabilitation therapies, their variation, and association with outcomes (Horn et al., 2015). This study provided the preliminary data used to design the CARE4TBI study.

Therapists at each site designed data collection forms to detail the interventions they conducted. They completed these forms in addition to standard clinical documentation, resulting in data with few gaps. Bogner emphasized the value of engaging providers in designing data collection tools, as people are more willing to dedicate time to capturing data that they deem useful. The CARE4TBI study uses the infrastructure of the NIDILRR-funded TBI Model Systems, and 14 of the TBI Model Systems sites are participating in CARE4TBI.

Multilevel stakeholder engagement is critical to the CARE4TBI process, said Bogner. For instance, the Ohio Valley Center Advisory Council (established in 1991) provides input on CARE4TBI and consists of individuals with TBI, advocates, and representatives from the rehabilitation field. Clinicians—including physicians; psychologists; and physical, occupational,

---

[2] See https://care4tbi.tbindsc.org/default.aspx (accessed January 3, 2024).

[3] Funded by NIDILRR, Bogner noted that the TBI Model Systems program is the world's largest TBI longitudinal database, with over 19,000 participants. For over 3 decades, TBI Model Systems has collected lifetime data on individuals with moderate to severe TBI from 16 inpatient rehabilitation sites. The TBI Model System National Data and Statistical Center provides the infrastructure required to manage a national database of this magnitude and hosts affiliated studies—such as CARE4TBI—enabling linked databases.

speech, and recreation therapists—have redesigned EHR formats to enable their use in research as well as program evaluation. From the outset, the CARE4TBI has been therapist driven, with therapists determining the key elements to capture in the study. Information technology (IT) specialists and EHR platform vendors collaborate in the initiative. Administration, such as rehabilitation leaders and upper hospital management, have enabled the study to effect change by allowing considerable changes within their systems.

Data Capture Standardization

The first phase of CARE4TBI focused on the standardization of EHR data capture, which involved identifying, designing, and standardizing data elements to be collected in session notes and ensuring these are extractable for both research and clinical operations. Bogner emphasized that data from EHR flow sheets are not necessarily extractable, thus flow sheets must be designed for data extraction. The CARE4TBI design considers efficiency for clinical operations by eliminating redundancy in existing data fields, aligning with regulatory requirements, and necessitating as few mouse clicks as possible. Once standardized, each rehabilitation site integrated the data fields into its existing workflow to maximize documentation efficiency. This means that all sites capture the same data elements, although the locations of these elements within the EHR may vary.

The design process prioritized ongoing collaboration with therapists and rehabilitation team leaders to create data elements aligned with therapists' priorities and a user-friendly data collection structure. IT professionals advised the design team on feasibility and ensured data extractability. The 2-year process of determining data elements and building templates concluded in August 2023. Fourteen sites integrated the templates into their workflow, trained clinical staff, and went live by September 2023. The data elements operate at various levels, with some fields completed at every session and others completed only when relevant. In accordance with medical record documentation standards, entries are limited to the content of sessions, and therapists are not prompted to indicate that an activity did not take place.

The standardization process faced numerous challenges, said Bogner. For example, hospital systems sometimes opt to share the cost of an EHR platform with other organizations. Although this method is effective in decreasing expenses, it reduces flexibility in customizing to a facility's preferences. For this reason, one site was unable to update the EHR and therefore discontinued participation in the study. Wider adoption of the CARE4TBI data elements within the rehabilitation field would enhance future data collection efforts, she said. The 14 sites that completed the first phase use two different EHR platforms—Epic and Cerner (major EHR vendors). Thus, the data elements design needed to accommodate both platforms as well as the various customizations that sites may select within each platform. To address this need, OSU built a template for the Epic platform that other sites using Epic could ingest. Each site using Cerner built its own template following CARE4TBI data elements guidance. The sites shared tips with one another to promote efficiency during this process. Additionally, some therapists prefer narrative notes to discrete fields such as dropdown menus. To facilitate the transition to structured, standardized fields, the design includes a comment section for each therapeutic activity. Terminology to describe the same activities varied between therapists. The study. made efforts to reach consensus on terminology and allowed for customization at the entry level to the extent that extraction reports remained consistent.

Data Collection and Analysis

Bogner reported that the second phase of CARE4TBI began on September 1, 2023, and will last for 5 years. This phase compares the effectiveness of various rehabilitation approaches in terms of community participation and the functional independence of patients with TBI. Furthermore, the study will identify patient, provider, setting, and postdischarge factors that modify the effect of therapy on outcomes. Researchers will use causal inference methods to analyze data on approximately 1,600 participants over the course of 5 years. Community participation and functional independence outcomes will be collected at discharge, 6 months postinjury, and 1 year postinjury.

TRACK-TBI NETWORK AND NINDS COMMON DATA ELEMENTS

Joseph Giacino, director of rehabilitation neuropsychology at Spaulding Rehabilitation Hospital and professor of physical medicine and rehabilitation at Harvard Medical School, discussed the Transforming Research and Clinical Knowledge in TBI (TRACK-TBI) study in terms of its aims, achievements, and efforts toward becoming a functioning LHS.[4] He began by identifying seven levels of care in the United States that—depending on the severity of the injury and length of the treatment course—may be appropriate for people with TBI.[5] He described this system as highly fragmented,

---

[4] More information about the TRACK-TBI network is available at https://tracktbinet.ucsf.edu/ (accessed November 30, 2023).

[5] These seven locations and levels of care are the emergency department, intensive care unit, acute care ward, inpatient rehabilitation hospital or long-term acute care hospital, skilled nursing facility, nursing home or other long-term care facility, and community- and home-based care.

lacking centralized management, and requiring navigation to successfully transition between the levels and locations of care; consequently, many people do not receive adequate TBI care and services. The LHS model offers care integration guided by research.

Learning Health System Components

Giacino outlined several components of an LHS for TBI, building on the 2022 National Academies' TBI report and 2006 IOM workshop. He highlighted the five areas of:

- Engaged Partnerships: Establishing an LHS requires engagement and close collaboration with diverse stakeholder groups, such as federal and state agencies that implement and regulate health service delivery, clinicians, payers, policy makers, individuals living with TBI, and caregivers. Partnerships with stakeholders identify common goals and well-defined roles.
- Harmonized Infrastructure: Harmonized infrastructure involves common data elements that apply to both research and clinical practice, EHR equipped with data capture, and data repositories with international interoperability.
- Standardized Data Acquisition: Standardized data acquisition features systematic, clinical data collection procedures that extend through all phases of recovery, particularly the postacute phase. Standardized outcome measures should be validated within specific contexts of use, such as diagnosis, prognosis, treatment efficacy, and patient stratification.
- Real-Tine Knowledge Access: Real-time access to curated knowledge can be made readily available to users via data visualization methods that facilitate interpretation (e.g., data dashboards) and decision support tools to guide care. Such tools should be easily accessible and meaningful to clinical practice.
- Continuous Learning Culture: A continuous learning culture is likely the defining feature of an LHS and is underdeveloped in the TBI field, he maintained. Such a culture requires LHS champions embedded in all sectors, sustainable education and training protocols, longitudinal assessment, and mechanisms to analyze and refine processes, such as feedback cycles.

These necessary—but not sufficient—LHS components enable a system that can answer questions related to diagnosis prognosis, and treatment, said Giacino. For example, a TBI LHS should be able to address diagnostic queries such as which performance-based TBI assessment measures can accurately detect mild TBI in adults within 48 hours postinjury. To support prognostication of anticipated recovery trajectory, the system should have the capacity to determine which TBI endophenotypes (subtypes), identified 1 month postinjury, indicate that a person is more likely to remain permanently dependent on others for activities of daily living. Such issues are particularly salient for patients and families as they envision their recovery process. Additionally, a TBI LHS should answer treatment questions such as which treatment is most effective for post-traumatic fatigue persisting longer than 12 weeks after a mild or moderate TBI. These examples highlight the specificity and relevance to patients that a TBI LHS should achieve, he said.

TRACK-TBI as a Learning Health System

A clinical trial network of 19 academic centers, TRACK-TBI features some of the foundational components of an LHS connecting research to care, Giacino said. The project focuses on four aims: (1) the creation of a legacy database to promote collaboration and accelerate TBI research, (2) improved TBI diagnosis and classification/taxonomy, (3) improved TBI outcome assessment, and (4) identification of the health and economic impact of mild TBI. A key objective is moving from the Glasgow Coma Scale (GCS) and Glasgow Outcome Scale to the adoption of a precision neuroscience approach that determines the endophenotypes of individuals with TBI through a combination of symptom reporting, multidimensional clinical data, neuroimaging, and blood-based biomarkers that inform personalized treatment.

Conceived as a public–private partnership, TRACK-TBI has established a diversely populated ecosystem of partners from industry, government, academia, and philanthropy over the past decade and has forged close ties to Europe's largest TBI study, the Collaborative European Neurotrauma Effectiveness Research in TBI (CENTER-TBI).[6] From the start, both projects have harmonized efforts and are using the NINDS TBI Common Data Elements to enable data sharing and, in turn, generate more robust research findings.[7] He noted that NINDS is creating a 3.0 version of the TBI Common Data Elements, and this version promises higher measurement precision than previous versions.

Given the variation in severity and symptom trajectory associated with TBI, TRACK-TBI needed a systematic assessment approach for a patient

---

[6] More information on CENTER-TBI is available at https://www.center-tbi.eu/ (accessed January 12, 2024).

[7] More information about the NINDS Common Data Elements is available at https://www.commondataelements.ninds.nih.gov/ (accessed November 30, 2023).

population with a level of function ranging from coma to uncomplicated mild TBI, said Giacino. Furthermore, the assessment must be able to accommodate the changes in level of function expected in the first year post-TBI. The study developed a flexible outcome assessment battery to systematically collect data on every participant at every time point regardless of the severity of impairment. TRACK-TBI has enrolled over 3,100 participants with TBI and more than 600 control participants, half of whom have orthopedic trauma and half of whom are friend controls. More than 3,000 data elements are collected per participant. The project has amassed over 3,200 adult MRI results taken at 2 weeks postinjury and 6 months postinjury to enable comparison. TRACK-TBI has acquired over 42,000 biospecimen samples (e.g., DNA, RNA, plasma, and serum) and performed over 3,200 follow-up exams with patients 2 to 8 years postinjury. This large dataset provides a critical foundation for analysis.

TBI Endpoints Development

Complementing TRACK-TBI and funded by the Department of Defense, the TBI Endpoint Development (TED) initiative created the TED metadataset by curating data from eight previous studies from the military, civilian, and sports sectors, Giacino explained.[8] The establishment of this metadataset allows for retrospective data mining in advance of conducting prospective studies. The initiative also conducted studies to validate selected common data elements within their context of use and then conformed these elements to global standards to facilitate data sharing and drug development.

TRACK-TBI Achievements

Giacino reviewed TRACK-TBI research findings and innovations to date, noting how the network's development of TBI-relevant clinical research tools, such as scoring and classification approaches, software modules, and data standards contribute to the underlying goal of linking research results to improved care through an LHS approach. Drawing on the network's array of tools and data, TRACK-TBI studies have demonstrated that deficits persist for at least 12 months postinjury in more than 50 percent of people who experience mild TBI (Nelson et al., 2019). Additionally, the risk of persistent functional impairment is highest for those with complicated mild TBI, meaning a TBI featuring a detectable structural lesion. On the other hand, over half of people who sustain severe TBI and

---

[8] More information about the TBI Endpoints Development initiative is available at https://tbiendpoints.ucsf.edu/ (accessed November 30, 2023).

remain severely disabled 2 weeks postinjury regain partial or full independence within 12 months (McCrea et al., 2021). He remarked that this finding undermines the pervasive nihilism about the prospects for recovery after severe TBI. Among the tools and technologies created via TRACK-TBI efforts, the Glasgow Outcome Scale-Extended (GOSE) is the outcome measure used most worldwide and is accepted by the U.S. Food and Drug Administration (FDA) for use in drug and device trials (Wilson et al., 2021).

This two-way scoring approach allows the investigator the flexibility to include peripheral injuries sustained by a patient in determining the disability rating or opt for a TBI-specific rating that discounts broken bones or other injuries that limit function. This differentiation is significant in determining disability severity, as a GOSE score that includes effects of peripheral injury will improve as peripheral injuries resolve. Although the studies launched at approximately the same time, TRACK-TBI uses the brain-specific outcome measure and CENTER-TBI uses the all-cause injury calculation. Without a mechanism to indicate the method being used, the CENTER-TBI outcomes would appear to be worse than those in TRACK-TBI. Thus, the integration of research was essential in delineating methods and understanding findings.

Additional TRACK-TBI developments include an evidence-based clinical outcome semiautomated Qualtrics platform that allows the validation of outcome measures within their specific context of use, said Giacino (Christoforou et al., 2020). The Clinical Data Interchange Standards Consortium incorporated the TRACK-TBI common data elements into the Therapeutic Area Data Standards in efforts to ensure global standardization (Clinical Data Interchange Standards Consortium, Inc., 2015). TRACK-TBI developed the OsiriX common data element software module, a standardized tool for evaluating MRI scans for TBI. This tool is used to identify imaging features associated with adverse outcomes after mild TBI and has been approved by the FDA for selecting mild TBI patients for clinical trials (FDA, 2019; Yuh et al., 2013, 2021). Most recently, a partnership with Abbott Labs, which developed the iStat Alinity point-of-care device, has enabled test results on TBI blood biomarkers within 15 minutes. Specifically, the glial fibrillary acidic protein (GFAP) and ubiquitin C-terminal hydrolase L1 (UCH-L1) proteins indicate whether a person has likely experienced a structural brain injury and therefore requires imaging (Yue et al., 2019).

TRACK-TBI Progress Toward LHS Realization

Giacino outlined a number of LHS components that TRACK-TBI has established, noting those that require additional efforts (see Figure 5-1).

In terms of engaged partnerships, he said, the project has brought together disparate stakeholder groups with common aims but needs to

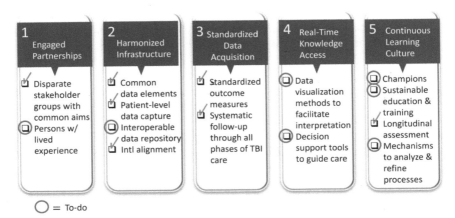

FIGURE 5-1 TRACK-TBI LHS scorecard.
NOTE: Areas achieved so far within the TRACK-TBI network are marked with red checks; green circles indicate areas in which further progress is needed.
SOURCE: Presented by Joseph Giacino, October 12, 2023.

deepen and expand partnerships with individuals with lived expedience of TBI. In working toward harmonized infrastructure, TRACK-TBI has made use of common data elements, patient-level data capture, and international alignment but has yet to establish an interoperable data repository. The network has successfully put the components of standardized data acquisition into place by developing standardized outcome measures and establishing systematic follow up through all phases of TBI care. Real-time knowledge access is currently lacking, given that the project has yet to develop data visualization methods to facilitate interpretation or decision support tools to guide care. Regarding cultivating a continuous learning culture, TRACK-TBI has established longitudinal assessment but has yet to engage additional champions of the effort, develop sustainable education and training, and build mechanisms to analyze and refine processes.

Giacino noted that the LHS components TRACK-TBI has not yet put in place constitute the difference between a system that achieves scientific advances and one that demonstrates real-world benefit from these advances. The former, for example, is capable of determining that a drug strikes a specified target, whereas the latter has the capacity to ascertain who actually takes the drug and whether it improves their health.

TRAUMATIC BRAIN INJURY DATA AND LEARNING SYSTEMS

Katharine Stout, assistant division chief at the Department of Defense (DoD) TBI Center of Excellence (TBICoE) noted that since 2000, over

479,000 service members have been diagnosed with at least one TBI (Figure 5-2) (DoD, 2023). She outlined two examples of DoD surveillance efforts intended to better understand TBI and translate these insights into an improved LHS. Long-range goals arising from this work include the creation of real-time dashboards built into the EHR to aid operational and medical leadership in improving clinical decision making and planning.

To inform awareness and measurement of TBI experienced by service members, DoD established a dataset of TBI occurrences, ICD codes, and approximations of when injuries occurred. Stout noted that DoD currently lacks the capability to track multiple TBIs experienced by a service member because of the International Classification of Diseases (ICD) coding structure used,[9] a barrier the department is working to address with partners across other agencies.

Stout shared several examples of how DoD TBI data have been used to inform medical monitoring, training, education. Leadership requested the

_____

[9] The International Classification of Diseases is a system for classifying medical conditions and used for such purposes as clinical record keeping, reimbursement of medical claims, and epidemiological surveillance. https://www.cdc.gov/nchs/icd/index.htm (accessed February 5, 2024).

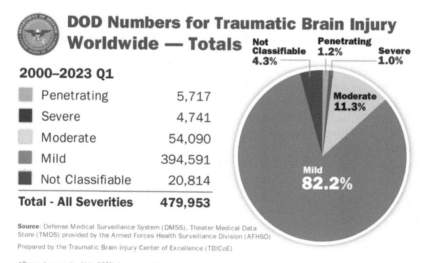

FIGURE 5-2 DoD traumatic brain injury totals as of May 9, 2023.
NOTE: Percentages may not add to 100 percent because of rounding.
SOURCE: Presented by Katharine Stout, October 12, 2023. Department of Defense (https://health.mil/Military-Health-Topics/Centers-of-Excellence/Traumatic-Brain-Injury-Center-of-Excellence/DOD-TBI-Worldwide-Numbers).

identification of military occupational specialties at higher risk for TBI. The analysis team cross-referenced service members identified with a first lifetime TBI between 2012 and 2019—numbering over 170,000—with DoD data systems containing occupation codes. Results indicated that Special Forces, Explosive Ordinance Devices units, and some artillery units were at a higher risk for TBI than other occupational specialties. The DoD regional educational coordinator network then targeted leadership in high-risk military occupational specialties to provide Warfighter Brain Health training to improve capacity for early TBI detection.[10]

Given that the DoD TBI case definition includes an "incidence rule" whereby service members only have one TBI counted per lifetime, Stout emphasized the need, and current efforts to establish, DoD surveillance methodologies to capture service members' subsequent TBIs. Additional areas to address include identifying service members who have already sustained multiple TBIs and creating management and treatment guidelines for such individuals. Within DoD, emergency medicine providers, first-line responders, rehabilitation providers, and nonmedical leadership have expressed interest and dedication in improving TBI treatment.

Constituting approximately 82 percent of service members diagnosed with TBI since 2000, individuals identified as having mild TBI demonstrate substantial variability in symptom presentation and trajectory, she said. The variety in TBI patterns, conditions, and symptoms poses challenges in triaging and triangulating care. Stout explained that this finding generated interest in improving the ability to identify patients with mild TBI and better predict their outcome trajectories. Both DoD and the Department of Veterans Affairs (VA) are currently working to introduce new data systems that connect to one another to improve the usefulness of the EHR for providers. TBICoE is examining how data from the system can be made actionable by prompting recommendations, treatment plans, and fact sheets for providers and making information available for patients with the aim of helping service members efficiently navigate treatment to return to their jobs and families to the greatest extent possible.

The surveillance team analyzes TBI data and reports on incidence, comorbidities, trends, and other results to inform military leadership (e.g., Agimi et al., 2018; Hai et al., 2023). A recent analysis described by Stout looked at comorbidities in military-sustained mild TBI by first identifying over 42,000 service members who experienced a first lifetime TBI between 2016 and 2019. Conducting a review of literature and TBI expert consensus, the surveillance team identified 18 conditions that often co-occur with mild

---

[10] More information at the Warfighter Brain Health Initiative is available at https://media. defense.gov/2022/Aug/24/2003063181/-1/-1/0/DOD-WARFIGHTER-BRAIN-HEALTH-INI-TIATIVE-STRATEGY-AND-ACTION-PLAN.PDF (accessed December 1, 2023).

TBI: alcohol and substance use disorders, anxiety disorders, cervicogenic disorders (e.g., perception of pain or dizziness arising from the neck), cognitive disorders, depression and other related conditions, headache and related conditions, hearing conditions, nausea/vomiting, neuroendocrine disorders, other neurological conditions, post-traumatic stress disorder (PTSD), other psychiatric conditions, psychological conditions, seizure-related conditions, sleep, suicidal and homicidal ideation, vestibular conditions, and visual disturbances. Stout highlighted the painstaking work involved in reviewing ICD codes and categorizing conditions. Researchers analyzed service member data records for conditions that were present 180 days prior to TBI diagnosis and those that appeared within the first 180 days postdiagnosis. She reported that over 77 percent of service members with mild TBI had at least one co-occurring condition, noting that 81 percent of the analyzed population were male, 64 percent were white, and 74 percent were younger than 34 years old. During the 180 days prior to TBI, the most frequently reported conditions were sleep-related conditions (21.7 percent), headache (19.4 percent), PTSD (17.8 percent), anxiety (11.3 percent), cervicogenic disorders (10.9 percent), and nausea/vomiting (7.7 percent). During the 180 days following mild TBI diagnosis, the prevalence of diagnosed conditions increased significantly, with visual disturbances and cognitive conditions increasing by over 300 percent, vestibular conditions increasing by 193 percent, headaches by 152 percent, and hearing-related conditions by 73 percent. Sleep-related conditions and anxiety disorders were moderately positively correlated with mild TBI. The period prevalence estimates of PTSD (30.1 percent) and depression and relation conditions (11.9 percent) among service members with mild TBI were higher than the 5 percent prevalence among nondeployed service members and 8 percent among combat deployment.

The findings confirmed anecdotal reports from providers, Stout said, and can aid in refining clinical recommendations and provider and patient education efforts. Given the busy schedules of care providers, information that offers clinicians specific symptoms to look for makes implementation of recommendations more manageable.

Stout also outlined several limitations to the findings. For example, conditions such as PTSD and suicidal ideation are likely underreported by service members because of associated stigma, and the presence of undiagnosed mild TBIs or other undiagnosed conditions could also contribute to underestimation of co-occurring conditions, particularly given that repeat TBIs are omitted by current DoD surveillance methodologies. Furthermore, assessment of service members with newly diagnosed mild TBI may uncover existing comorbid conditions not related to TBI. Additional efforts are needed to further understand the interplay of comorbid conditions to enhance provider ability to triage, treat, and move patients through the appropriate trajectory of care.

DISCUSSION

Developments in Care, Research, and Learning Integration

Umoh asked about advances that have been achieved in TBI treatment and recovery through integrated linkages between care, research, and continuous learning. Bogner replied that foundational work for CARE4TBI identified some approaches most likely to effectively improve outcomes. Implementing these approaches does not necessitate changes to the natural rehabilitation environment, she said, but rather a shift in emphasis. For example, when therapists perform activities relevant to daily life with patients during inpatient sessions, patients are more likely to resume normal activities outside of the home 1 year postinjury than when therapists focus on clinic-based activities. She stated her hope that CARE4TBI will generate more nuanced guidance as the project moves forward.

Giacino noted two initiatives underway that can contribute to the further development of TBI LHSs. He noted the TBI forum's ongoing action collaborative on TBI care. Members of the action collaborative are currently focused on fostering and disseminating best practices, care models, and more integrated care systems for people with suspected TBI who are released from the emergency department (ED). These individuals may not be connected to any follow up care, although many experience ongoing symptoms. Additionally, the Biomedical Advanced Research and Development Authority is conducting an aid-in-diagnosis trial to validate the use of blood-based biomarkers for TBI detection. How to establish LHS feedback loops and iterative learning as these and other advances move into clinical application will require future consideration, he noted. Beth McQuiston, neurologist, dietitian, and medical director of diagnostics at Abbott Laboratories, noted that this aid-in-diagnosis trial is being conducted in partnership with Abbott to study TBI biomarkers used on a core laboratory platform, which would also integrate into a system's EHR for use in assessing TBI severity level.

Stout described a DoD instruction that represents a paradigm shift for service members with acute concussion or potentially concussive events who are being discharged from the ED or from "sick call," the military equivalent of urgent care. Rather than instructing patients to follow up for care if certain symptoms present, the policy specifies a follow-up visit within 72 hours. This practice enables early identification of TBI patients who become symptomatic after the initial care visit. Aligning with the Military Acute Concussion Evaluation 2 and Progressive Return to Activity Following Acute Concussion tools,[11] this policy represents a substantial change

---

[11] For these tools, see https://health.mil/Reference-Center/Publications/2020/07/30/Military-Acute-Concussion-Evaluation-MACE-2 and https://health.mil/Reference-Center/Publications/2023/01/23/Progressive-Return-to-Activity-Primary-Care-for-Acute-Concussion-Management (accessed January 12, 2023).

in practice and has met some challenges in implementation. For instance, clinic schedules require flexibility to allow for follow-up visits within 3 days. TBICoE is working closely with medical affairs at the Defense Health Agency to refine the policy and its metrics.

Another forthcoming paradigm shift involves moving from a pre-deployment mandate for neurocognitive assessment testing to assessment over the lifetime of a service member. This shift is expected to improve assessment accuracy and collect objective measures on service members that generate real-time data. In developing the capacity to rapidly use findings to aid service members in returning to full duty to the greatest extent possible after TBI, this development can move the system toward full realization as an LHS.

Challenges in Establishing a Learning Health System

Two substantial challenges in shifting DoD toward becoming an LHS are behavior change and adoption of new tools, Stout asserted. The department is using feedback loops to address these challenges. For example, practitioners in the field expressed the desire for greater accessibility of the tools than the current PDF format. TBICoE is working with IT to house the tools within a mobile application and make it possible to download the tools onto mobile devices to use when wireless Internet service is unavailable. This format will increase ease of use within the clinical setting. Additionally, efforts are underway to integrate the tools into the EHR to increase adoption in the clinic and enable data capture. This change will move away from text paragraph fields to radio buttons to allow providers to indicate a patient's symptoms and functional levels without typing. This development is intended to decrease provider time spent on documentation and increase data capture fidelity. She emphasized that soliciting and acting upon feedback from stakeholders improves practice, generates better data, and opens communication. Bogner noted a past challenge in assessing implementation, as CARE4TBI issued recommendations to therapists but lacked data on adoption. Use of the standard data fields generates practice data that inform implementation assessment. Establishing the ability to rapidly receive data and translate it into a visual format that clinical providers can use in decision making is a current challenge.

Lessons Learned

Highlighting the complexity of large systems, Bogner noted her surprise at the heterogeneity in electronic health record platforms across different sites. Additionally, much of the documentation that providers enter into the EHR is aimed at supporting clinical use but is not provided in a format that can be evaluated to improve clinical operations and outcomes across an organization and system. Current data at most rehabilitation facilities are merely a record of the treatment that occurred and cannot be used for program evaluation or examining outcomes, she said. Many sites have done little more than transfer paper forms into electronic systems, and thus most electronic health systems have yet to collect data in a format that can be used to improve patient outcomes. Stout noted the challenge of creating systems that effectively capture outcomes, aggregate data from multiple datasets, and provide real-time data to clinicians in a format that improves care. Current data are disjointed and do not offer providers a clear navigation path. Using a football analogy, she said that improving the TBI "playbook" for providers would increase their ability to become "star quarterbacks" who help patients navigate to best possible outcomes.

Giacino remarked that building improved infrastructure will enable access to better care. The knowledge gained over the past decade eclipses that of the 30 years prior, he said, and technology and data sharing between large networks can accelerate the learning process. He emphasized the importance of including all stakeholders as LHS initiatives are designed. Describing TRACK-TBI as slower to incorporate patients up front in development, he underscored the critical value of lived experience and also stated that engagement of payers is key in LHS discussions and the creation of new payment models.

TBI Prevention

Kristine Yaffe, director of the Center for Population Brain Health at the University of California, San Francisco, asked how an LHS can improve prevention efforts, given the high rates of PTSD and sleep impairment prior to TBI and that a prior TBI constitutes the biggest risk factor for experiencing another TBI. For example, a data dashboard could potentially assess TBI risk similar to fall-risk calculations for older adults. Bogner stated that prevention is critically important and must start with primary care providers. Stout remarked that TBI prevention efforts should extend within medical operations and beyond the health care system to the education system. Work conducted on exposure risk via section 734 of the National Defense Authorization Act for Fiscal Year 2018 led the military operational and safety communities to issue a safety memorandum regarding the TBI risk posed by blast exposure.[12] Efforts are underway to determine a definitive marker for TBI on blast gauges.

In the meantime, the safety memo states that service members with exposure to pressure greater than 4 pounds per square inch should be con-

---

[12] National Defense Authorization Act for Fiscal Year 2018, Public Law 115-91, 115th Cong., 1st sess., (December 12, 2017).

sidered at high risk for a potentially concussive event. She emphasized that this guidance was an operational initiative, rather than a medical one. Prevention efforts for TBI could resemble those for diabetes, in which standard annual physical exams include the hemoglobin A1C test—an early marker for diabetes—and a certain A1C level triggers diabetes education efforts. Given the broad nature of TBI as a medical condition and its intersections with, for example, occupational safety issues, TBI prevention necessitates participation of communities beyond medical and rehabilitation professionals, said Stout.

Culture Change

Corinne Peek-Asa, vice chancellor for research at University of California, San Diego, asked about opportunities and challenges involved in structural and cultural change. Giacino remarked on the difficulty of shifting culture and noted he is beginning a grant-funded implementation project focused on culture change. Identifying what constitutes an LHS champion, who these champions are, and how they will function is important to cultural transformation, he said. This change process requires a mechanism to ensure that change efforts are ongoing and sustained. Such a mechanism involves human resources, which come at a cost. However, his review of literature indicates that efforts that do not aim for culture change from an initiative's start are likely to fail. Focus groups can be used within the TBI field to better understand the barriers and facilitators to care encountered by patients and caregivers. Incorporating the perspective of end users into the system design can shift culture to better meet the needs of individuals with TBI.

Emergency Medical Services TBI Data

Bruce Evans, immediate past president of the National Association of Emergency Medical Technicians, remarked that the National Emergency Medical Services Information System database is not relational to other health care databases. Thus, data collected by emergency medical services (EMS) on TBI patient encounters are not connected to Epic or other EHR databases and undermine the ability to perform longitudinal assessments. Moreover, EMS can directly affect the cost of TBI care, particularly if EMS providers deliver a patient to the wrong level of trauma care, discharge the patient, or allow a patient to become hypotensive, hypothermic, or hypoxic. He asked how databases can be better connected to improve longitudinal assessment. Bogner replied that the TBI Model Systems program performs lifetime tracking of TBI patients who receive inpatient rehabilitation services.

Currently, the program is monitoring individuals 35 years postinjury. In the past, TBI Model Systems datasets included EMS data; however, this was ended because of the issues Evans raised. She described the disconnection between EMS data and other medical system databases as problematic, disrupting the ability to conduct long-term follow up on all TBI patients who receive EMS care. Stout commented on the variety of data systems across DoD environments and roles of care. An effort is currently underway to aggregate data, but legacy systems present challenges with variance in data fields and data fidelity. Giacino noted that probabilistic matching techniques can be used to match identical patients within two separate databases that do not communicate. The National Traumatic Databank and TBI Model Systems conducted probabilistic matching with some success, he said.

Payment Models for TBI Care

Giacino underscored the challenge of integrating an LHS with payment models. Many people in the United States receive excellent acute care for TBI and then encounter a care gap after discharge. Many people with a moderate-to-severe TBI do not receive comprehensive inpatient rehabilitation services, he said. Those who do receive this care are typically limited to 19 days of inpatient rehabilitation, and many people are discharged in an acute state of confusion. Noting the programs for postacute care in Massachusetts that have been shut down because of lack of funding, he emphasized that best practice will only be implemented if supported by payment models.

Donald Berwick, president emeritus and senior fellow of the Institute for Healthcare Improvement, raised the possibility of constructing payer structures to propose to the payer community that would outline needed changes, the patients' needs that such changes would meet, and cost. He asked about the feasibility of this approach. Giacino remarked that rehabilitation services are limited by a "3-hour rule" from the Centers for Medicare and Medicaid Services (CMS). This rule limits the authorization of admission to inpatient rehabilitation to individuals who are able to actively participate in rehabilitation services for 3 hours per day. However, the neurobiology of severe TBI often does not allow that level of activity. Commercial payers often impose the limits set by CMS. He noted that his institution abides by this rule because of payment ramifications, and that it impedes access to care for many TBI patients, particularly those who require inpatient rehabilitation after discharge from the acute care hospital. Addressing such barriers could increase access to needed care.

Bogner commented that little to no evidence supports the 3-hour rule. Research indicates that the content of the therapy and extent to which the participant engages is responsible for improved TBI outcomes, rather than a specified time spent participating. Giacino commented that talks with commercial payers about the benefits of even limited participation in inpatient rehabilitation for TBI patients have stalled once cost entered the discussion.

Odette Harris, professor of neurosurgery at Stanford University and deputy chief of staff for rehabilitation at the Veterans Affairs Palo Alto Health Care System, stated that cost is central in treatment coverage. Given that VA is not bound by the restrictions set by CMS, the requirement of 3 hours active participation has been lowered at some VA polytrauma sites because of the lack of evidence supporting clinical relevance of this threshold on outcomes. However, when cost implications come into play, blame is often attributed to those who made the determination to offer the rehabilitation services. She added that a comparison of patients who meet the threshold for the 3-hour rule and those who do not failed to reveal any differences in outcome. Geoffrey Manley, chief of neurosurgery at San Francisco General Hospital and vice chair of neurological surgery at University of California, San Francisco, emphasized that many patients will be unable to access the interventions they need to fully return to their families and jobs without changes to this 3-hour rule.

John Corrigan, director of the Ohio Valley Center for Brain Injury Prevention and Rehabilitation, commented that the Forum on Traumatic Brain Injury should address insurance-related barriers and could look to other countries in doing so. For example, Australia and New Zealand do not rely solely on health insurance to cover costs and have spread financial responsibility to accident insurance. Payment model reform would benefit government sources, given that individuals with poor TBI outcomes are more likely to require government assistance in the forms of Medicaid and Medicare.

TBI Classification

Berwick noted that the National Academies of Sciences, Engineering, and Medicine's 2022 TBI report indicated that categorizing TBIs as mild, moderate, and severe could impede insights to progress (NASEM, 2022). He asked whether efforts to move away from this categorization method are still deemed necessary. Bogner replied that the current classification system does a disservice to individuals who sustain TBI. Regardless of whether the terms *mild*, *moderate*, and *severe* are used, an improved TBI classification system could extend beyond a medical model to incorporate the effects of environment and community on a patient's ability to recover. This shift would acknowledge that outcomes are not only affected by the extent of injury, but also by the supports an individual can access during recovery.

Manley remarked that during patient interviews across the country, patients and families shared that they do not want the "mild, moderate, and severe" labels used. Some family members refused early withdrawal of life-sustaining therapies for their loved ones with severe TBI, and now those patients have not only survived, but have returned to work. Others were labeled by the ED as having mild TBI and have since been unable to work. Thus, this terminology can create bias in expected outcomes. In January 2024, NINDS hosted a workshop on TBI classification and nomenclature that examined the current classification system and considered factors beyond the biology on the day of injury—reflected in GCS score, blood-based biomarker level, and computerized tomography scans—to factors in the biological, psychological, social, and environmental model. Echoing Bogner, he noted that biology at injury does not dictate outcome trajectory. Rather, factors including social setting, environment, treatment interventions, and qualification for rehabilitation services form a complex web that affects outcome and thereby requires a comprehensive approach to TBI care and recovery.

6

Data Capture, Surveillance, and Supporting Long-Term Care Needs

Key Points Highlighted by Individual Speakers[1]

- Most traumatic brain injury (TBI) burden estimates are generated from hospital data, resulting in rates that skew toward severe TBI and underestimate the true prevalence of TBI. (Daugherty)
- The Centers for Disease Control and Prevention's National Concussion Surveillance System pilot survey found that 12 percent of adults and 10 percent of children reported experiencing a head injury in the past year, representing significant increases from prevalence rates in other studies. (Daugherty)
- The 2023 and 2024 National Health Interview Surveys now feature five questions on TBI and provide national-level surveillance data. (Daugherty)
- State registry data can be used to better understand state-level TBI rates, but usage guidelines vary by state and data are limited to individuals who visit the hospital. (Miller)
- Lack of interoperability poses a barrier to synthesizing data from numerous and varied sources collecting data on individuals with TBI. (Miller)

---

[1] This list reflects the rapporteurs' summary of points made by the identified speakers, and the statements have not been endorsed or verified by the National Academies of Sciences, Engineering, and Medicine. They are not intended to reflect a consensus among workshop participants.

- Virginia is conducting TBI screening efforts in community-based services such as domestic violence and mental health programs to fill data gaps. (Miller)
- Efforts to standardize questions included on state surveys could facilitate a better understanding of the nationwide effects of TBI. (Miller)
- Sheltering Arms Rehabilitation Centers monitor and collect data on all practices, analyze data to increase intervention effectiveness, and track and assist individuals after services end to improve outcomes. (Miller)
- The risk for numerous conditions increases with TBI, such as sleep disorders, cardiovascular disease, cancer, accidents, suicide, and homicide. (Hoffman)
- The Department of Veterans Affairs is working to improve TBI outcomes by exploring and developing multimodal TBI biomarkers, improving screening and evaluation methods, and evaluating a multidisciplinary care approach for potential scaling. (Hoffman)

The sixth session of the workshop focused on national, state-level, and agency data analysis efforts to inform public health and patient care strategies. It spotlighted programs by the Centers for Disease Control and Prevention (CDC), the Virginia Department for Aging & Rehabilitative Services (DARS), and the Department of Veterans Affairs (VA) to collect surveillance data, collaborate with community partners, and ultimately improve outcomes for individuals living with traumatic brain injury (TBI). Kristine Yaffe, director of the Center for Population Brain Health at the University of California, San Francisco; Rebeccah Wolfkiel, executive director at the National Association for State Head Injury Administrators; and Corinne Peek-Asa, vice chancellor for research at University of California, San Diego, served as moderators of the session.

TRAUMATIC BRAIN INJURY SURVEILLANCE AT CDC

Jill Daugherty, epidemiologist on the CDC Division of Injury Prevention TBI Team, discussed the agency's TBI surveillance efforts, including how such data informs development of the National Concussion Surveillance System. The CDC TBI team has four prioritized goals: (1) identify effective strategies to prevent youth sports- and recreation-related TBI, (2) identify and test methods to improve the measurement of TBI burden, (3) characterize TBI-related disparities and identify strategies to increase health equity, and (4) determine effective strategies to improve the diagnosis and management of TBI. Highlighting the second goal, she explained that CDC efforts to better understand the public health burden of TBI include conducting surveillance, monitoring trends in TBI incidence and prevalence, and identifying groups disproportionately affected by TBI. Surveillance aids in the development of specialized TBI interventions and in the detection of disproportionate disease burden. Moreover, TBI surveillance increases the understanding of the most common principal mechanisms of injury and informs creation of mechanism-based TBI prevention efforts.

National Concussion Surveillance System Pilot

Historically, the CDC TBI team has used health care datasets to conduct surveillance work, said Daugherty. These data indicate that approximately 214,000 TBI-related hospitalizations took place in the United States in 2020 (CDC, 2023). In 2021, approximately 69,000 TBI-related deaths occurred. Although TBI-related hospitalizations have decreased each year that CDC has documented these data, deaths have slowly increased. These figures constitute a substantial public health problem, yet they do not capture individuals with TBI who sought care in a primary care or urgent care setting or did not seek care. Hence, TBI burden data are skewed toward more severe TBIs that require hospitalization or cause death and underestimate the true prevalence of TBI in the United States. Over the past decade, CDC has worked to establish a National Concussion Surveillance System (NCSS) to address this issue.

Daugherty described that a 2014 National Academies consensus study, *Sports-Related Concussions in Youth: Improving the Science, Changing the Culture*, outlined gaps in incidence and prevalence estimates of youth sports-related concussion and recommended that CDC establish and oversee a national surveillance system to accurately determine the incidence of sports-related concussion in youth (IOM-NRC, 2014). Congress indicated support for the NCSS via the TBI Program Reauthorization Act of 2018, which stated that CDC may implement concussion data collection and analysis to determine the prevalence and incidence of concussion.[2] However, it was not until December 2022 that Congress made a budget appropriation for concussion surveillance. The CDC TBI team designed and fielded an NCSS pilot in 2018 and 2019 with the primary goals of testing methodology and evaluating a novel TBI case definition for use in classifying TBI based on self-report data.

---

[2] Traumatic Brain Injury Program Reauthorization Act of 2018, Public Law 115-377, 115th Cong., 2d sess. (December 21, 2018).

Methodology featured a household survey administered via computer-assisted random digit dial telephone survey. The pilot study interviewed adults about head injuries that they or their children sustained in the previous 12 months, and adolescents aged 13 to 17 years were interviewed separately. Researchers collected information on signs and symptoms experienced after each head injury, participant demographics, mechanism of injury—including whether the injury was sports related—medical care received, and indicators of postinjury functioning. Data collection launched in September 2018 and concluded 1 year later after obtaining completed surveys on approximately 10,000 adults, 3,500 children ages 5 to 17 years by proxy reporting from their parents, and 198 adolescents.

Preliminary conclusions of the NCSS pilot data indicate that 12 percent of adults and 10 percent of children reported experiencing a head injury in the prior year, constituting higher percentages than found in other surveys, said Daugherty. Given that the pilot was established to fill data gaps on individuals who do not receive medical treatment in a hospital setting following injury, researchers expected that prevalence rates would surpass those of other studies.

After conducting the survey, she said, researchers determined the pilot study was overly complex. The survey included questions regarding up to three head injuries the adult experienced and up to three head injuries per child for up to seven children in the household. In households with high burden, the survey became excessively lengthy, highlighting the need for a streamlined collection tool. Additionally, the sample size of 198 adolescents was much smaller than that of younger children and of adults owing to the difficulty in gaining consent to interview adolescents directly.

Next Steps in Establishing National Surveillance

Proposed NCSS next steps include an address-based sampling methodology to survey randomly selected adults about head injuries sustained in the previous 12 months, Daugherty said. Researchers plan to make the survey less burdensome by only inquiring about the most recent head injury that adult respondents or their children sustained. Furthermore, respondents will have the option of completing the survey by telephone call-in or online. The pilot generated a revised TBI case definition, and this will serve as the basis for incidence and prevalence estimates. CDC has awarded a contract for the next iteration of NCSS, which will use a modified survey based on pilot results.

Expanding the Knowledge Base

A continuously operating NCSS would increase the TBI knowledge base by providing national prevalence and incidence estimates of TBI in the United States, Daugherty said. Ongoing surveillance would identify the most common mechanisms of TBI, which may differ from the mechanisms that result in hospitalization or mortality. Surveillance data could deepen the understanding of TBI outcomes in terms of common symptoms, the amount of time missed from work or school as a result of injury, and whether medical evaluation was sought. Furthermore, researchers could use NCSS data to identify those who are at a higher risk of sustaining a TBI. Given that fully establishing the NCSS will take time, CDC is concurrently laying groundwork for the NCSS while using alternate methods of surveillance. For example, the CDC TBI team added five questions to the 2023 National Health Interview Survey.[3]

Conducted by the CDC National Center for Health Statistics, this survey has been collecting data with a large sample size for several decades. Two of the five added questions pertain to TBI prevalence, two ask about sports- and recreation-related TBI, and one question regards medical evaluation after injury. The 2024 survey will repeat these questions and will provide national-level TBI surveillance data, although these data will lack the granularity of the NCSS pilot survey.

Additionally, the CDC Behavioral Risk Factor Surveillance System (BRFSS) gathers nationally representative data via an annual survey.[4] The survey content varies by state, and TBI questions are not part of the core survey, precluding the generation of nationally representative data on TBI. Although some states have opted to include modules for TBI, the questions vary by state and data cannot necessarily be easily combined nor compared. The CDC TBI team is working to increase adoption of optional TBI modules among additional states to expand the state-level TBI data available. She noted that BRFSS data are released approximately 8 months after data collection, demonstrating CDC's commitment to delivering timely data for public health action.

DEVELOPING LEARNING HEALTH SYSTEMS
TO SUPPORT LONG-TERM CARE NEEDS

Christiane Miller, director of the DARS Brain Injury Services Coordination (BISC) Unit, focused on the key roles that state-level data and community-based services play in care once patients leave the hospital, and discussed efforts in Virginia to collect and integrate data from a variety of sources—including community service providers—to better understand

---

[3] More information about the National Health Interview Study is available at https://www.cdc.gov/nchs/nhis/index.htm (accessed December 5, 2023).

[4] More information about the Behavioral Risk Factor Surveillance System is available at https://www.cdc.gov/brfss/index.html (accessed December 5, 2023).

outcomes and improve supports for people with TBI. The Virginia Department of Health (VDH) uses registry data for outreach and other needs. In collaboration with the Brain Injury Association of Virginia, BISC sends outreach letters to all people identified by the trauma-specific registry as having a TBI. In 2022, letters sent to 160 individuals resulted in only a 3 percent response rate. However, individuals with TBI sometimes respond to the letters more than a year later, stating that they did not follow up sooner because of being overwhelmed after their injury.

Guidelines vary from state to state in terms of limits to data registry access and whether multiple outreach efforts are allowed. Additionally, statutes for registries are not funded in all states, and thus not all states have registries. In Virginia, registry data are underused and are only now being explored for uses beyond outreach, said Miller. Hospitals are required to upload data to the VDH database on a quarterly basis. Over the past decade, the participation rate of hospitals completing the majority of data elements has increased dramatically. Given that these data contain demographic and geographic information and the first point of hospital discharge, mining the registry data and combining it with other sources could create a more complete and accurate picture of TBI in Virginia.

Miller emphasized that registry data are sourced from hospitals and therefore do not include individuals unless they visit the emergency department for their head injuries. Access to registry data often becomes available 3 to 6 months postdischarge. However, this delay appears to coincide with the amount of time many patients need to feel ready to respond to outreach efforts.

TBI Model Systems Collaboration

Virginia houses a TBI Model Systems site at Virginia Commonwealth University (VCU), said Miller. The state allocates trust fund revenues—generated from a portion of the fees collected at driver's license reinstatement—to research and implementation of new or innovative services. In 2018, the Virginia DARS contracted with the VCU TBI Model System to develop a plan for integrating the data resources that could be used to plan and expand services for people living with TBI. After a search for all possible TBI-related databases and resources, the VCU TBI Model System explored four specific data sources: the Virginia state trauma registry; the Virginia All-Payer Claims Database (APCD), the Rehabilitation Services Administration Case Service Report (RSA-911), and TBI Models Systems data. Researchers collected data on the use of inpatient and outpatient treatment from APCD, data on employment outcomes for students graduating from high school from RSA-911, and approximately 35 years of long-term outcomes data from TBI Model Systems. Thus far, efforts to integrate these datasets have been unsuccessful because of the lack of common identifiers. In recent years, Virginia has developed a data trust, and this may prove useful in the future.

Miller said that the lack of connected data systems led to the Virginia Brain Injury Data Sharing Summit in 2022, at which brain injury professionals, service providers, and state agency representatives convened to discuss ways forward. Among the needs highlighted at the summit, a better understanding of where people with TBI receive community-based services outside of the TBI system was identified as necessary for facilitating connections and collaborations needed to effectively collect and use TBI data. For example, domestic violence programs, jails, department of corrections, homelessness programs, and mental health programs often interact with individuals with TBI, and screening conducted at such sites could fill data gaps. Furthermore, the summit identified the need to better understand TBI comorbidities and other co-occurring challenges in order to develop training, screening, and collaborative services for TBI clients who also face issues related to mental health, substance use disorder, intellectual or developmental disabilities, housing, employment, and/or aging.

Currently, a Virginia-wide TBI screening effort is taking place in domestic violence programs, and three pilot programs in homeless shelters will soon begin implementation. Additionally, a federal grant-funded pilot screening program will be conducted in at least two community-based mental health programs and one state mental health facility. She emphasized the importance of designing sustainable efforts and embedding these into the processes of all agencies and stakeholder groups.

Next Steps in Virginia TBI Data Collection

Following the initial research project and data summit, a second 3-year trust fund grant was awarded to the VCU TBI Model System to research transitions and disparities in care and outcomes for neurotrauma, said Miller. This work will identify when and how transitions of care occur, how these transitions affect outcomes, and those at greater risk of experiencing negative health outcomes. Moreover, BISC is working to gather data via the BRFSS. As Daugherty mentioned, BRFSS survey content varies by state. Currently, Virginia does not have approval to include optional questions, but BISC is completing an application to gain approval to add TBI-related queries to the data collection effort. She noted that the ability to glean TBI data from the BRFSS survey would not only benefit Virginia, it would contribute to a clearer picture of the nationwide effects of TBI. These data could potentially inform treatment, advocacy, policy, and funding. Cost for the BRFSS varies across states and can be prohibitive. She raised the idea of TBI experts collaboratively identifying a set of questions and advocating for their addition to the BRFSS in each state. Such an effort would enable the comparison of outcome indicators such as health status, number of healthy days, health care access, exercise, and alcohol consumption.

Virginia uses state funds to purchase case management, day support, and other related services from eight community-based brain injury service providers, Miller described. Historically, the data required from these providers has been limited to the numbers of clients served and their demographic information. Efforts are currently underway to collect data on outcomes, which would aid in identifying services that are most effective and areas that need more support. The state could then direct funding with more precision. On January 1, 2024, Virginia amended its state plan to include Medicaid reimbursement for targeted brain injury case management services. This development comes after a year of preliminary work with the Virginia Department of Medical Assistance Services. Prior to this collaboration, BISC lacked state-level data on individuals with TBI from Medicaid health care claims and on services provided via developmental disability Medicaid waiver.[5] The effort to establish Medicaid reimbursement for brain injury services opened a trove of data to BISC; the unit plans to analyze data from Medicaid, managed care organizations, and state-funded providers to identify outcomes.

Sheltering Arms Rehabilitation Centers

Miller described Sheltering Arms Rehabilitation Centers as an example of a learning health system (LHS). In partnership with the VCU TBI Model System, Sheltering Arms collects and uses data to evaluate the effectiveness of their practices and protocols. Monitoring extends to all practices, including those identified as evidence-based best practices, to determine the effectiveness of processes and interventions with different individuals. Sheltering Arms works to identify differences in effectiveness stemming from specific individual needs or intervention delivery. Recognizing that the challenges individuals face do not disappear once services end, this data-based organization established a care transitions program in which community health workers track patients for 6 to 12 months to provide information and to help ensure that patients are attending medical appointments and taking prescribed medications. She noted that these services resemble transition-of-

---

[5] States request Medicaid waivers from the Centers for Medicare and Medicaid Services (CMS). Waiver programs allow states to provide covered home- and community-based services and supports to qualifying individuals. Information on such waiver programs is available at https://www.medicaid.gov/medicaid/home-community-based-services/home-community-based-services-authorities/home-community-based-services-1915c/index.html. Information on Virginia's Developmental Disabilities waiver program is available at https://www.dmas.virginia.gov/for-providers/long-term-care/waivers/ (accessed February 26, 2024).

care services for older adults moving from inpatient to outpatient settings. A TBI Model Systems grant will enable community health workers to engage with caregivers to determine needed supports. Miller commented on the invaluable insight gleaned from direct communication with individuals with TBI and their caregivers, and she urged researchers to routinely engage in dialogue with TBI survivors, even if only on an annual basis, to gain perspective on aspects of living with the injury that may not emerge from the data.

LEARNING HEALTH SYSTEMS FOR TRAUMATIC BRAIN INJURY IN THE VA

Stuart Hoffman, senior health science officer for TBI for the VA Office of Research and Development, discussed VA efforts to better understand TBI comorbidities, develop TBI multimodal biomarkers, improve screening and evaluation efforts, and identify and scale effective treatment approaches. He outlined that an LHS involves systems of leadership, governance, community building, research, data and analytics, and quality improvement (Lannon et al., 2021). Leadership encourages a network to perform as a system, governance directs research, community building forms connections between investigators and clinicians, and research and data analytics inform improvements in health care services and generate innovation.

Causes of TBI in service members include training, shoulder-fired weapons, and occupational blast, and often involve repetitive exposures, Hoffman explained. He recounted an exchange years ago with a veteran receiving care at the Defense and Veterans Brain Injury Center—now the Traumatic Brain Injury Center of Excellence—who was diagnosed with a TBI while being treated for a limb injury. When Hoffman asked about the TBI, the veteran said that his challenges stemmed from post-traumatic stress disorder (PTSD), not TBI. This gave him pause, as the veteran was receiving care at a brain injury center and not at a mental health treatment facility. He began to consider the various treatment destinations for veterans with TBI, including mental health services, neurology providers, and physical medicine and rehabilitation. Additionally, some individuals who enter the armed forces are at a higher risk for TBI. For example, rural areas are overrepresented in TBI prevalence data. Approximately a third of veterans with a lifetime history of TBI experienced their first TBI before the age of 18. The complexity of TBI led Hoffman to look to an LHS as a mechanism for exploring comorbidities.

TBI Comorbidities

A 2009 study of 340 veterans returning from service in Iraq found high co-occurrence rates of persistent postconcussive symptoms, PTSD, and chronic pain (Lew et al., 2009). Hoffman explained that at that time, an understanding of TBI's complexity was beginning to emerge. Up to that point, some mental health professionals believed that any brain injury–related disability lasting longer than 30 days should be attributed to a mental health issue rather than TBI. Care providers now know that in some cases TBI symptoms last for years and often co-occur with conditions such as sensory disorders; psychological conditions including PTSD, depression, substance use disorder, and suicidal ideation; chronic pain; mobility issues; cognitive disorders; executive dysfunction; effort control impairment; and endocrine dysfunction. A 2021 study of nearly 200,000 VA electronic health records (EHRs) found that, after adjusting for demographics and medical and psychiatric conditions, veterans with TBI were 41 percent more likely to develop a sleep disorder than veterans without TBI (Leng et al., 2021). He emphasized that poor sleep quality affects health, mental health, and quality of life.

Having TBI increases one's risk of cardiovascular disease (CVD), and both TBI and CVD are risk factors for dementia, said Hoffman (Kornblith et al., 2022). Moreover, veterans with TBI have higher mortality rates from accidents, suicide, cancer, CVD, and homicide than veterans without TBI and the general population (Howard et al., 2022). Suicide rates are 57 percent higher for veterans than for nonveterans, and TBI exacerbates this risk (Howard et al., 2023). Increased impulsivity associated with TBI can fuel behaviors that create dangerous situations; this dynamic may account for the higher homicide mortality rate seen among veterans with TBI. He noted that an upcoming paper examines an increased risk for certain cancers associated with moderate, severe, and penetrating brain injury. The increased risk of mental and physical health problems for people with TBI shortens lives and may also play a role in the increased risk of suicide in this population, he added.

Biomarkers Research, Screening, and Evaluation

The Commander John Scott Hannon Veterans Mental Health Care Improvement Act of 2019 includes a requirement via section 305 that VA fund an initiative to identify, validate, and integrate brain and mental health biomarkers among veterans, Hoffman said.[6] The requirement launched the Precision Mental Health for Veterans Initiative, which uses longitudinal studies to meet the intent of the law and develop multimodal biomarkers

---

[6] Commander John Scott Hannon Veterans Mental Health Care Improvement Act of 2019, Public Law 116-171, 116th Cong., 2d sess. (October 17, 2020).

using imaging, assessments, fluid markers, and physiological measures. The longitudinal studies come from the Long-term Impact of Military-relevant Brain Injury Consortium—Chronic Effects of Neurotrauma Consortium (LIMBIC-CENC) and the Translational Research Center for TBI and Stress Disorders (TRACTS). A partnership between VA and DoD, LIMBIC-CENC is a federally funded research project to better understand, treat, and prevent TBI.[7] This project follows a cohort of veterans and service members broken into subgroups: TBI, TBI in addition to a mental health condition, a mental health condition and no TBI, and a control group. Based in Boston, TRACTS is a Rehabilitation Research and Development National Center for TBI Research that features long-term chronic TBI populated cohorts and has been operating for over a decade.[8] The Precision Mental Health for Veterans Initiative is working to integrate biomarker measures into a clinical, actionable diagnostic.

Current VA data collection efforts include screening and a comprehensive evaluation of veterans from Operation Enduring Freedom, Operation Iraqi Freedom, and Operation New Dawn, said Hoffman (Figure 6-1). However, approximately one-third of veterans are not participating in the evaluation despite repeated requests. He stated that possible causes for lack of participation include difficulty remembering the evaluation, attributing symptoms to a comorbid condition rather than to TBI, or having difficulty engaging because of depression. To improve the participation rate, VA is developing a telemedicine approach to the comprehensive evaluation. Furthermore, VA is evaluating a multidisciplinary care approach for veterans with TBI to streamline access to neurological care, physical rehabilitation services, and mental health care.

The VA Quality Enhancement Research Initiative is currently evaluating this multidisciplinary approach. Should it prove successful, this approach will scale from five current sites to 23 network sites, with potential scaling to other VA sites nationwide. Additionally, a longitudinal study focusing on veterans with mild TBI is underway, and an upcoming longitudinal study will examine the trajectories of veterans with severe TBI. Hoffman emphasized that ongoing communication with clinicians enables researchers to understand treatment needs, and the resulting research generates findings that inform clinicians of best practices.

---

[7] More information about the Long-term Impact of Military-relevant Brain Injury Consortium—Chronic Effects of Neurotrauma Consortium is available at https://www.limbic-cenc.org/ (accessed December 6, 2023).

[8] More information about the Translational Research Center for TBI and Stress Disorders is available at https://www.va.gov/boston-health-care/research/the-translational-research-center-for-tbi-and-stress-disorders-tracts/ (accessed December 6, 2023).

Consistent Identification of TBI

Current Opportunity

- Identifying Veterans with TBIs can help to **inform clinical providers to properly assess Veterans** who are at most risk for various physical and mental health conditions

Infrastructure Needs

Funding for developing and implementing a **virtual comprehensive evaluation** for TBI to improve rate identification

TBI Interdisciplinary Care

- The **complex comorbidities** associated with TBI require interdisciplinary care
- Upon completion of QUERI evaluation for IETP, **implementation research** will focus on the next level of Polytrauma Network sites

The next phase will be to **scale this program to network sites** through investment and research focus on how to create interdisciplinary outpatient capabilities

Longitudinal Study of Mild to Severe TBI

- There remains a **gap for severe TBI progression**, especially regarding disorders of consciousness
- Currently, these Veterans are **cared for at skilled nursing facilities, at home by family, or lost to follow**

Building on existing infrastructure of the Long-term Impact of Military-relevant Brain Injury Consortium (LIMBIC) effort; in addition, build a **system to track Veterans with severe TBI** to better understand the progression of condition to improve care.

FIGURE 6-1 Examples of how the Department of Veterans Affairs is using research infrastructure and integration with clinical care to support better outcomes for veterans with TBI.
NOTE: IETP = Intensive Evaluation and Treatment Program; QUERI = VA Quality Enhancement Research Initiative.
SOURCE: Presented by Stuart Hoffman, October 12, 2023.

DISCUSSION

Incidence Estimate Factors

Given that the NCSS pilot study reported higher incidence numbers than estimates in previous studies, Ramon Diaz-Arrastia, director of the TBI Clinical Research Center at the University of Pennsylvania, asked whether trivial head impacts might account for the variance. Daugherty acknowledged the possibility that minor head injuries that would not be classified as TBIs in a clinical setting were included in the incidence estimate. To address this, the study is using a tiered case definition that uses reported signs and symptoms to distinguish between a "probable TBI" and a "possible TBI." For instance, a head injury with the sole symptom of headache would be classified as a possible TBI. This distinction will enable researchers to divide cases according to "probable" or "possible" TBI classification before prevalence and incidence estimates are published. Thereby, a more conservative estimate will include only the probable TBIs, such as people with head injuries who lost consciousness, have post-traumatic amnesia, or experience other specific symptoms.

Cases with more general symptoms that are not necessarily indicative of TBI would then be excluded from conservative estimates. She added that she is unaware of a national TBI incidence estimate that includes people who did not seek medical attention. The inclusion of people who experienced head injuries but were not seen in a health care setting could account for the discrepancy between the 12 percent of adults estimated to have experienced a TBI in the NCSS pilot study and the lower estimates in other studies. The 2017 Youth Risk Behavior Surveillance system estimated that 15 percent of high school students reported a past-year concussion from participating in sports (DePadilla et al., 2018). She noted that estimates from studies based solely on health care databases or that are not nationally representative are difficult to compare with NCSS pilot study estimates.

Data Collection Funding Sources

Wolfkiel asked about funding sources for the data collection mechanisms used in Virginia. Miller explained that the Virginia General Assembly funds these research efforts, enabling DARS to dedicate trust fund dollars to other areas. She noted that states without general assembly-allocated funds sometimes opt to use trust funds for research. A grant from the Administration for Community Living (ACL) funds the screening pilot programs that will soon be implemented in homeless shelters and community- and facility-based mental health providers. A prior ACL grant enabled the VCU

TBI Model System collaboration that explored data sharing and led to the Virginia Brain Injury Data Sharing Summit.

TBI Screening of High-Risk Populations

Wolfkiel asked Miller to discuss the role of screening and the use of screening data in service provision. Community screening enables the identification of people with TBI in non-health care settings, Miller replied. For example, a screening project conducted a few years ago in the juvenile justice system found that almost 50 percent of participants were at risk of having TBI. She expects that the screening program used by homelessness service providers will yield similar results for people experiencing homelessness. Individuals who had not experienced a TBI at the onset of homelessness may be at an increased risk of head injury because of the lack of safety associated with being unhoused. Many states are also exploring TBI screening in domestic violence programs because of the increased TBI risk from exposure to violence. In addition to data collection, screening efforts increase awareness of TBI among the service providers working with populations at higher risk for TBI, she emphasized. The screening programs involve training for community service providers and partners these organizations with local, community-based brain injury programs.

To facilitate TBI screening, the National Association of State Head Injury Administrators (NASHIA) launched the Online Brain Injury Screening and Support System (OBISS), an online, cloud-based version of the Ohio State University TBI Identification Method.[9] The screening tool's online format can be used in a variety of settings. With this tool in place, BISC can recommend screening implementation to the community-based mental health centers they communicate with. The screening results can then inform training needs. Miller remarked that BISC had allocated almost $100,000 to the process of incorporating a screening tool into the EHR. The advent of OBISS made it possible to instead purchase a subscription for the screening tool and reallocate remaining funds to other needs. During intake, staff can review the OBISS results and indicate in the EHR when an individual is at risk of having TBI. The EHR can then trigger referral processes for therapists and case management teams. Simultaneously, this system provides BISC with state-level OBISS data.

Social Factors as Complex Causes of TBI

Given the current political unrest and major disasters affecting many of the world's continents, traumatic stress and biomechanical traumatic

---

[9] See https://www.nashia.org/obisssprogram (accessed January 12, 2024).

injury will likely increase, Peek-Asa noted. She asked how systems might approach integrating factors such as biochemical sequelae of psychological trauma and biomechanical, cellular, and physical damage to neurons and brain structures. Hoffman replied that this complex interplay warrants care from integrative, multidisciplinary care teams, such as the teams in place at the Palo Alto, San Antonio, Tampa, Richmond, and Minneapolis VA Polytrauma Rehabilitation Centers. Transferring this care approach to the private sector would likely require a payment algorithm that enables insurer coverage for these services.

Telemedicine in Patient Engagement

Referencing the third of veterans who screened positive for TBI but did not respond to requests to participate in a comprehensive evaluation, Jeffrey Bazarian, University of Rochester Medical Center, asked whether telemedicine is effective in increasing engagement in evaluation. Hoffman noted that currently, VA telemedicine evaluations are in the planning stages as a component of a validation study. A group from the VA Hudson Valley health care system has been conducting telemedicine evaluations on a smaller scale for several years and has seen positive outcomes from this effort. Thus, VA is looking at scaling this approach and determining the feasibility of having staff available to answer calls for evaluations 24 hours a day, 7 days a week.

The Role of Medicaid Waivers in the TBI Care System

Donald Berwick, president emeritus and senior fellow of the Institute for Healthcare Improvement, asked about the status of state Medicaid waivers for TBI, whether a template or model waiver is available to aid additional states in implementation, and how many states are currently providing this eligibility status to individuals with TBI. As noted by Miller, state Medicaid waivers that enable longer term home- and community-based services and supports are an important aspect of the care ecosystem for many people impacted by TBI, highlighting how the learning health system concept for TBI needs to extend beyond hospital-based systems.

Miller noted that there are multiple options for TBI-relevant waivers, including community-based waivers and pilot demonstration waivers. John Corrigan, director of the Ohio Valley Center for Brain Injury Prevention and Rehabilitation, stated that approximately 19 states currently have TBI Medicaid waivers in place. The variance between waivers reflects a lack of standardization that may warrant consideration of creating a template or model. However, a general trend away from additional population-specific Medicaid waivers is at play, and some states have recently incorporated

TBI-specific waivers into more generic disability waivers. Miller also shared her experience in seeking a TBI Medicaid waiver in Virginia, which has not yet been approved. The process of demonstrating feasibility and obtaining approval for new waivers is often complex. In Virginia, for example, efforts to obtain a TBI waiver have involved the state Medicaid agency as well as colleagues from NASHIA and technical assistance funds from CMS.

State-Level Surveillance Data

Peek-Asa asked about opportunities to incorporate state-based TBI surveillance into plans for a nationally weighted data sample. Daugherty remarked on the feedback received from states on the value of state-level TBI prevalence and incidence estimates. A potential opportunity to meet the needs for both nationally representative estimates and state-level estimates involves creating NCSS on a scale large enough to produce both state and national estimates. This would necessitate expanding NCSS by an approximate magnitude of 20 in terms of sample size and resources needed. Although such a development would not take place for several years, the possibility of obtaining representative samples from each state is being considered, she said. A second option is to use BRFSS by adding TBI questions to the core survey. In the event that changing the core survey is not feasible, NCSS could create a standardized module that states could adopt to enable state-to-state comparisons. She noted that states currently must opt in to include TBI questions on customized BRFSS surveys. CDC is exploring the feasibility of various approaches to generating both state- and national-level TBI surveillance data.

Hoffman called for advocacy toward a national act for TBI similar to the National Alzheimer's Project Act, which increased treatment and research for Alzheimer's disease (AD).[10] Given that a greater number of people in the United States are experiencing lingering TBI symptoms than AD-related dementia, and that a portion of individuals with AD likely had one or more TBIs in their lifetime, TBI warrants increased services, funding for better care, and more research, he contended.

---

[10] National Alzheimer's Project Act, Public Law 111-375, 111th Cong., 2d sess. (January 4, 2011).

7

Using Learning Health Care Systems to Combat Inequitable Outcomes in Traumatic Brain Injury

Key Points Highlighted by Individual Speakers[1]

- Partnerships with community-based partners can raise awareness of traumatic brain injury (TBI), increase services to individuals with TBI via bidirectional referrals, and facilitate screening efforts. (Reisher)
- Programs targeting assistance to youth and to older adults provide needed support, but working-age individuals may encounter a services gap. (Reisher)
- Screening efforts in populations at high risk for TBI revealed that a sizeable majority of participants in domestic violence programs, youth detention, and mental health programs had likely experienced a brain injury. (Reisher)
- Community-based service providers are often unaware of the high risk for TBI within the populations they serve and lack an understanding of how TBI can affect behavior, decision making, and participation. (Reisher)

---

[1] This list reflects the rapporteurs' summary of points made by the identified speakers, and the statements have not been endorsed or verified by the National Academies of Sciences, Engineering, and Medicine. They are not intended to reflect a consensus among workshop participants.

• A trauma-informed care approach is appropriate for individuals with TBI, yet awareness is lacking about the need for such an approach with the TBI population. (Reisher)

The seventh session of the workshop explored community partnerships as a mechanism to identify populations at a higher risk for traumatic brain injury (TBI), to expand TBI screening, and to build system capacity, particularly in areas with less access to TBI specialty care. Monique Pappadis, associate professor at the University of Texas Medical Branch at Galveston, moderated the session.

MEETING CLIENT NEEDS AND ENHANCING COMMUNITY CAPACITY

Peggy Reisher, executive director of the Brain Injury Alliance of Nebraska (BIA-NE), discussed the organization's efforts to partner with community programs to estimate TBI burden, raise awareness, and provide services to individuals living with TBI. While working as a social worker in the TBI unit at Madonna Rehabilitation Hospital, she observed the limited services available to people once they leave the hospital. This service gap inspired her to collaborate in establishing BIA-NE, a statewide nonprofit organization working toward the mission of creating a better future for all Nebraskans through brain injury prevention, education, support, and advocacy. Serving individuals with TBI and acquired brain injury, BIA-NE provides services free of charge and does not require proof of brain injury. The organization has 10 employees to cover the entire state, much of which is rural, and places a particular focus on high-risk populations. Client support services include resource facilitation—linking clients to community support services—and brain injury–specific education.

Noting that some clients never visit the hospital for their brain injuries, she explained that individuals may not have accessed any brain injury education or services before contacting BIA-NE. In an effort to address the limited services and supports available for people with brain injuries in Nebraska, BIA-NE works to build systems capacity. Resource facilitators educate and collaborate with community providers, offering information and guidance about brain injury screening and case management. BIA-NE created a public service announcement video to generate awareness about the education and consultation services available to community providers.

Nebraska Brain Injury Data

In addition to providing resource facilitation, education, and capacity-building services, BIA-NE collects data on brain injuries in Nebraska, said Reisher, noting that many brain injury alliances and associations collect similar data and could offer insight within the context of partnerships to address TBI. In data BIA-NE has captured since July 1, 2021, 627 clients experienced 821 brain injuries, with leading causes including motor vehicle crashes (21 percent), falls (12 percent), nondomestic assault (12 percent), and domestic violence (9 percent). Among current BIA-NE clients, 80 percent of 749 injuries were TBIs and 20 percent were injuries stemming from internal health events or injuries less severe than TBI. The client average age at time of injury is 31 years old, with individuals ranging in age from 0 to 88 years old. She emphasized that some community-based programs provide support to children and adolescents with brain injury while others focus on older adults, but a services gap often exists for working-age individuals.

Referrals and Resource Facilitation

The majority of referrals to BIA-NE come from nonhospital sources, Reisher noted. Unfortunately, many clients do not hear about the organization until years after their injuries. Among BIA-NE clients served from July 2022 to June 2023, 24 percent received services within a year of their most recent injury, 19 percent began services 1 to 2 years postinjury, 18 percent received services within 3 to 5 years, and 39 percent did not receive resource facilitation services until more than 5 years after their injuries. She underscored that these numbers are an improvement from prior years, which she attributes to the organization's public awareness efforts. Currently, two BIA-NE employees work closely with a corrections facility in Nebraska, resulting in increased referrals. Indeed, corrections constitutes the largest BIA-NE referral source, generating 16 percent of total referrals. Other leading referral sources include Internet searches (13 percent), community-based organizations (13 percent), and friends or family (12 percent). Only 6 percent of BIA-NE referrals come from hospitals.

Ongoing outreach efforts to community-based organizations have fueled an increase in referrals from these service providers. The most common area of need for clients is education about brain injury and how to best contend with its effects. Many of the staff members have experienced a brain injury themselves or have a loved one with a brain injury, enabling them to provide a personal perspective. In fact, Reisher works to hire staff with personal experience for this reason. Resource facilitators refer BIA-NE clients to a variety of service providers, with 30 percent of referrals made to community-based organizations. A substantial proportion of clients, perhaps as many as half, have never been seen by a medical professional for their brain injuries and therefore require referrals to primary care providers or specialists. In sum, BIA-NE refers clients to 112 different organizations for needs ranging from medical care to housing to transportation. The organization also provides informational materials to clients.

Building Systems Capacity for High-Risk Populations

Many individuals with TBI do not receive services specific to brain injury, Reisher emphasized. However, some such individuals are involved with the Department of Behavioral Health, corrections, domestic violence programs, and other services. To better support people with brain injuries, BIA-NE has focused its efforts on populations at high risk to increase identification and connection to appropriate services. A grant-funded project that provided brain injury screening in domestic violence programs found that 58 percent of clients likely had TBI. Reisher described that such screening efforts also serve as a mechanism for raising awareness among program staff. For instance, during screening implementation, employees working at domestic violence programs made comments such as "Oh, maybe that's why she doesn't show up" and "Maybe that's why she looks like she doesn't care." In response, BIA-NE facilitators discuss the difference between clients who *won't* comply with program requirements and those who *can't*, helping staff members to recognize the difference between deficit and defiance. A recent approval of a National Institutes of Health Research Project Grant (R01) will enable the implementation of brain injury screenings to a greater number of domestic violence programs in Nebraska.

Similar efforts are underway for youth in juvenile detention programs, said Reisher. Currently, BIA-NE is conducting screening with youth detained at the Douglas County Youth Center, the largest juvenile detention facility in Nebraska. Using a version of the Ohio State University TBI Identification Method (OSU TBI-ID) screening tool modified to include questions about acquired brain injury, BIA-NE screening efforts indicate that 67 percent of youth detained at the facility had likely experienced a brain injury. The organization is also conducting screening in mental health programs. At one behavioral health center, 77 percent of individuals screened positive for brain injury. She noted that many of the staff at mental health programs, including psychologists and psychiatrists, respond to BIA-NE training as if the brain injury information is new to them. The organization is currently working to establish a contract with an inpatient state hospital to screen patients at behavioral health hospitals.

Reisher explained that screening does not equate to brain injury diagnosis, and that facilitators make this clear during the training and the screening process. In addition to the OSU TBI-ID, screeners at the juvenile detention center use a juvenile symptoms questionnaire developed by the Mindsource Brain Injury Network.[2] This tool captures symptoms related to memory, processing, attention, inhibition, physical and sensorimotor, language, organization, mental flexibility, and emotions. In comparing results of the symptoms questionnaire with those from the OSU TBI-ID, statistical differences emerge between those who have likely experienced a brain injury and those who have not. Reisher noted concern from some participating programs, particularly within juvenile justice, that participants will use the information learned from screening as an excuse for problematic behavior. In reply, BIA-NE recommends that programs use the information learned from population screening and implement trauma-informed care practices to address needs related to brain injury. The organization provides management strategies to programs to use in working with clients with behaviors that may be related to deficits.

Training and Data Gaps

Many medical professionals in Nebraska do not have a thorough understanding of brain injury, and brain-injury specific training for medical professionals could benefit patients, Reisher said. To address patient information needs, BIA-NE has been working with some providers to cobrand brain injury-specific handouts to provide to patients at medical appointments or upon hospital discharge. She noted that providers appear more open to providing cobranded materials to patients than materials from BIA-NE. Training is also needed for community providers, and partnerships with state- or national-level brain injury alliances and associations can be used to meet this need. Currently, 10 state programs affiliated with the Brain Injury Association of America or the U.S. Brain Injury Alliance are using cloud-based software from Salesforce, Inc., to collect client data on cause of injury, gender, and race/ethnicity. Moving forward, the potential exists to add areas of need to this data collection. Each state organization is independent, and therefore the data from these 10 states are not connected. Reisher stated that assistance in examining data across states could benefit medical professionals as well as state organizations.

---

[2] The Mindsource Brain Injury Network juvenile symptom questionnaire is available at https://mindsourcecolorado.org/juvenile-symptom-questionnaire/ (accessed December 9, 2023).

DISCUSSION

Awareness Gaps

Pappadis asked about current gaps in TBI awareness for service providers and for individuals living with TBI. Reisher remarked on a tendency among service providers to blame individuals for behaviors that are related to brain injury. She lauded the growing awareness of trauma-informed care and stated that the exclusion of brain injury information from trauma-informed care training is to the detriment of social justice. Some researchers have resisted BIA-NE requests to include brain injury in their studies, citing the absence of a concrete biomarker and the difficulty in differentiating whether certain behaviors should be attributed to brain injury or to other conditions such as attention-deficit/hyperactivity disorder. Given that limits within health insurance coverage often result in shortened hospital stays—and that many people experience brain injury symptoms for a long period of time—people with brain injuries often require community-based services, she noted. Providers of these services need additional training to better understand clients with brain injury, she said.

John Corrigan, director of the Ohio Valley Center for Brain Injury Prevention and Rehabilitation, remarked on the endorsement of trauma-informed care within behavioral health, domestic violence, and other systems of care. He explained that trauma-informed care is not a specific treatment, but rather knowledge and awareness that extreme emotional distress, particularly when experienced during childhood, can affect behavior years later. Similarly, neurologic-informed care is the awareness that neurologic impairment can affect behavior, helping providers to distinguish between *can't* and *won't*. Set for publication in November 2023, the American Society of Addiction Medicine Criteria guidelines on levels of care for substance use disorder treatment will include a chapter on cognitive impairment. It introduces the term *neurologic-informed care* and states that all people, regardless of subtle or obvious cognitive impairment, should be treated at every level of care for substance use disorder. He commented on the current opportunity to increase the understanding of brain injury and its behavioral implications within the community system.

Medical School Curriculum

Reisher commented that more information about brain injuries should be included in education for medical students. She shared her surprise at being asked to speak about brain injury at a webinar for medical professionals, given her expectation that medical professionals would already be well informed about brain injury. Presenting prevalence data on risk groups, she encouraged the webinar attendees to be particularly mindful that patients who have experienced domestic violence, homelessness, or detainment in the criminal justice system are at a high risk for having sustained a brain injury. Corrigan noted discussions with the U.S. Medical Licensing Examination organization about the content of the exam in regard to brain injury. He was informed that exam questions about brain injury are limited to examples of concussion and do not include more severe brain injury. James Kelly, professor of neurology at the University of Colorado School of Medicine, stated that during the Barack Obama presidential administration, Michelle Obama and Jill Biden launched the Joining Forces initiative to better meet the needs of service members and veterans. That initiative convened approximately 60 deans of medical schools to discuss areas including improved training for TBI treatment. Despite voiced commitments to modifying the curriculum to better address TBI, limited changes have been made.

Similarly, a group of representatives from the Association of American Medical Colleges, the American Medical Association, and the American Nurses Association gathered under the auspices of the Joining Forces initiative. Meeting monthly for over a year, the group made commitments to influence curriculum change to better address brain injury within the education for their various specialty areas. However, the traction of this effort appears to have been lost, said Kelly.

Rural Considerations

Reisher underscored the difficulty of accessing brain injury–specific care in a rural state such as Nebraska. Only one neuropsychologist who understands brain injury practices within an area comprising approximately two-thirds of the state. This makes obtaining a neuropsychological assessment challenging. She expressed hope that access to telemedicine will help to close this gap in the future. Noting that services are often more limited in rural versus metro areas, she emphasized that capacity building is needed in all locations to effectively meet the needs of individuals with brain injury.

WORKSHOP WRAP-UP

Corinne Peek-Asa, vice chancellor for research at the University of California, San Diego, recapped how the workshop featured an exploration of multiple levels and elements involved in developing a learning health system (LHS). Opening with the lived experience of Lindsay Simpson, cofounder of the Champion Comeback Foundation, the workshop moved from the individual patient experience to opportunities to pilot test and then to quickly scale and translate findings into improved treatment for patients.

In her talk, Simpson described contending with the effects of TBI and the challenges and barriers she has encountered in accessing effective treatment. Giving a charge to the audience to address some of these barriers, Peek-Asa noted that innovation is a pathway to accelerate solutions to patient problems, and the workshop showcased examples of feasible, low-cost methods of introducing innovation to processes. She emphasized that LHSs should center on patient needs and opportunities.

Communication systems should routinely be built into practice to facilitate smoother patient navigation experiences, increase caregiver engagement, and foster collaboration with primary care and other providers, Peek-Asa continued, emphasizing that core LHS principles provide guidance in improving systems and aligning continuous improvement areas. Speakers during the workshop discussed change efforts ranging in scale from large federal initiatives to modifying a health system's electronic health record. Sessions explored the roles of payer engagement and culture change in establishing sustainable improvements in treatment and care delivery.

Illustrative examples of LHS activity described during the workshop demonstrated how partnership, integration, translation, capacity, and scaling enable accelerated problem solving, Peek-Asa said. Surveillance can inform the understanding of TBI burden, trends, and risk factors, and a multilevel LHS can bolster health equity and health justice by ensuring that every decision moves toward better care, better prevention, better treatment, and better recovery for all, she said. Donald Berwick, president emeritus and senior fellow of the Institute for Healthcare Improvement, closed by spotlighting the importance of and movement toward cooperation evident in the TBI field's willingness to work together to improve care and outcomes for individuals with TBI.

A

References

Agimi, Y., L. E. Regasa, B. Ivins, S. Malik, K. Helmick, and D. Marion. 2018. Role of Department of Defense policies in identifying traumatic brain injuries among deployed US service members, 2001-2016. *American Journal of Public Health* 108(5):683-688.

CDC (Centers for Disease Control and Prevention). 2023. *Traumatic brain injury and concussion.* https://www.cdc.gov/traumaticbraininjury/index.html (accessed December 5, 2023).

Christoforou, A. N., M. J. Armstrong, M. J. G. Bergin, A. Robbins, S. A. Merillat, P. Erwin, T. S. D. Getchius, M. McCrea, A. J. Markowitz, G. T. Manley, and J. T. Giacino. 2020. An evidence-based methodology for systematic evaluation of clinical outcome assessment measures for traumatic brain injury. *PLoS One* 15(12):e0242811.

Clinical Data Interchange Standards Consortium, Inc. 2015. *Therapeutic area data standards user guide for traumatic brain injury version 1.0 (provisional).* Austin, TX: Clinical Data Interchange Standards Consortium, Inc.

CMS (Centers for Medicare and Medicaid Services). 2023. NHE Fact Sheet. https://www.cms.gov/data-research/statistics-trends-and-reports/national-health-expenditure-data/nhe-fact-sheet (accessed February 9, 2024).

DePadilla, L., G. F. Miller, S. E. Jones, A. B. Peterson, and M. J. Breiding. 2018. Self-reported concussions from playing a sport or being physically active among high school students—United States, 2017. *MMWR Morb Mortal Wkly Rep* 67(24):682-685.

DoD (Department of Defense). 2023. *DoD TBI worldwide numbers.* https://health.mil/Military-Health-Topics/Centers-of-Excellence/Traumatic-Brain-Injury-Center-of-Excellence/DOD-TBI-Worldwide-Numbers (accessed December 1, 2023).

FDA (U.S. Food and Drug Administration). 2019. *FDA in brief: FDA takes new step to help advance the development of novel treatments for traumatic brain injury with the qualification of a medical device development tool.* https://www.fda.gov/news-events/fda-brief/fda-brief-fda-takes-new-step-help-advance-development-novel-treatments-traumatic-brain-injury (accessed November 30, 2023).

Hai, T., Y. Agimi, and K. Stout. 2023. Prevalence of comorbidities in active and reserve service members pre and post traumatic brain injury, 2017–2019. *Military Medicine* 188(1-2):e270-e277.

Horn, S. D., J. D. Corrigan, J. Bogner, F. M. Hammond, R. T. Seel, R. J. Smout, R. S. Barrett, M. P. Dijkers, and G. G. Whiteneck. 2015. Traumatic brain injury-practice based evidence study: Design and patients, centers, treatments, and outcomes. *Arch Phys Med Rehabil* 96(8 Suppl):S178-S196.e115.

Howard, J. T., I. J. Stewart, M. Amuan, J. C. Janak, and M. J. Pugh. 2022. Association of traumatic brain injury with mortality among military veterans serving after September 11, 2001. *JAMA Network Open* 5(2):e2148150-e2148150.

Howard, J. T., I. J. Stewart, M. E. Amuan, J. C. Janak, K. J. Howard, and M. J. Pugh. 2023. Trends in suicide rates among post-9/11 US military veterans with and without traumatic brain injury from 2006–2020. *JAMA Neurol* 80(10):1117-1119.

IOM (Institute of Medicine). 2000. *To err is human: Building a safer health system*. Edited by L. T. Kohn, J. M. Corrigan, and M. S. Donaldson. Washington, DC: National Academy Press.

IOM. 2001. *Crossing the quality chasm: A new health system for the 21st century*. Washington, DC: National Academy Press.

IOM. 2007. *The learning health care system: Workshop summary*. Edited by L. Olsen, D. Aisner, and J. M. McGinnis. Washington, DC: The National Academies Press.

IOM. 2015. *Vital signs: Core metrics for health and health care progress*. Edited by D. Blumenthal, E. Malphrus, and J. M. McGinnis. Washington, DC: The National Academies Press.

IOM-NRC (Institute of Medicine-National Research Council). 2014. *Sports-related concussions in youth: Improving the science, changing the culture*. Edited by R. Graham, F. P. Rivara, M. A. Ford, and C. M. Spicer. Washington, DC: The National Academies Press.

Kornblith, E., A. Bahorik, Y. Li, C. B. Peltz, D. E. Barnes, and K. Yaffe. 2022. Traumatic brain injury, cardiovascular disease, and risk of dementia among older US veterans. *Brain Inj* 36(5):628-632.

Lannon, C., C. L. Schuler, M. Seid, L. P. Provost, S. Fuller, D. Purcell, C. B. Forrest, and P. A. Margolis. 2021. A maturity grid assessment tool for learning networks. *Learn Health Syst* 5(2):e10232.

Leng, Y., A. L. Byers, D. E. Barnes, C. B. Peltz, Y. Li, and K. Yaffe. 2021. Traumatic brain injury and incidence risk of sleep disorders in nearly 200,000 US veterans. *Neurology* 96(13):e1792-e1799.

Lew, H. L., J. D. Otis, C. Tun, R. D. Kerns, M. E. Clark, and D. X. Cifu. 2009. Prevalence of chronic pain, posttraumatic stress disorder, and persistent postconcussive symptoms in OIF/OEF veterans: Polytrauma clinical triad. *J Rehabil Res Dev* 46(6):697-702.

McCrea, M. A., J. T. Giacino, J. Barber, N. R. Temkin, L. D. Nelson, H. S. Levin, S. Dikmen, M. Stein, Y. G. Bodien, K. Boase, S. R. Taylor, M. Vassar, P. Mukherjee, C. Robertson, R. Diaz-Arrastia, D. O. Okonkwo, A. J. Markowitz, G. T. Manley, O. Adeoye, N. Badjatia, M. R. Bullock, R. Chesnut, J. D. Corrigan, K. Crawford, A. C. Duhaime, R. Ellenbogen, V. R. Feeser, A. R. Ferguson, B. Foreman, R. Gardner, E. Gaudette, D. Goldman, L. Gonzalez, S. Gopinath, R. Gullapalli, J. C. Hemphill, G. Hotz, S. Jain, C. D. Keene, F. K. Korley, J. Kramer, N. Kreitzer, C. Lindsell, J. Machamer, C. Madden, A. Martin, T. McAllister, R. Merchant, L. B. Ngwenya, F. Noel, A. Nolan, E. Palacios, D. Perl, A. Puccio, M. Rabinowitz, J. Rosand, A. Sander, G. Satris, D. Schnyer, S. Seabury, M. Sherer, A. Toga, A. Valadka, K. Wang, J. K. Yue, E. Yuh, and R. Zafonte. 2021. Functional outcomes over the first year after moderate to severe traumatic brain injury in the prospective, longitudinal TRACK-TBI study. *JAMA Neurol* 78(8):982-992.

NAM (National Academy of Medicine). 2023. *Emerging stronger from COVID-19: Priorities for health system transformation*. Washington, DC: The National Academies Press.

NASEM (National Academies of Sciences, Engineering, and Medicine). 2022. *Traumatic brain injury: A roadmap for accelerating progress.* Edited by D. Berwick, K. Bowman, and C. Matney. Washington, DC: The National Academies Press.

Nelson, L. D., N. R. Temkin, S. Dikmen, J. Barber, J. T. Giacino, E. Yuh, H. S. Levin, M. A. McCrea, M. B. Stein, P. Mukherjee, D. O. Okonkwo, C. S. Robertson, R. Diaz-Arrastia, G. T. Manley, O. Adeoye, N. Badjatia, K. Boase, Y. Bodien, M. R. Bullock, R. Chesnut, J. D. Corrigan, K. Crawford, A. C. Duhaime, R. Ellenbogen, V. R. Feeser, A. Ferguson, B. Foreman, R. Gardner, E. Gaudette, L. Gonzalez, S. Gopinath, R. Gullapalli, J. C. Hemphill, G. Hotz, S. Jain, F. Korley, J. Kramer, N. Kreitzer, C. Lindsell, J. Machamer, C. Madden, A. Martin, T. McAllister, R. Merchant, F. Noel, E. Palacios, D. Perl, A. Puccio, M. Rabinowitz, J. Rosand, A. Sander, G. Satris, D. Schnyer, S. Seabury, M. Sherer, S. Taylor, A. Toga, A. Valadka, M. J. Vassar, P. Vespa, K. Wang, J. K. Yue, and R. Zafonte. 2019. Recovery after mild traumatic brain injury in patients presenting to US Level I trauma centers: A transforming research and clinical knowledge in traumatic brain injury (TRACK-TBI) study. *JAMA Neurol* 76(9):1049-1059.

NIH Panel (National Institutes of Health Consensus Development Panel on Rehabilitation of Persons with Traumatic Brain Injury). 1999. Rehabilitation of persons with traumatic brain injury. *JAMA* 282(10):974-983.

Shrank W. H., T. L. Rogstad, and N. Parekh. 2019. Waste in the US health care system: Estimated costs and potential for savings. *JAMA* 322(15):1501-1509.

Wilson, L., K. Boase, L. D. Nelson, N. R. Temkin, J. T. Giacino, A. J. Markowitz, A. Maas, D. K. Menon, G. Teasdale, and G. T. Manley. 2021. A manual for the Glasgow Outcome Scale-Extended Interview. *J Neurotrauma* 38(17):2435-2446.

Yue, J. K., E. L. Yuh, F. K. Korley, E. A. Winkler, X. Sun, R. C. Puffer, H. Deng, W. Choy, A. Chandra, S. R. Taylor, A. R. Ferguson, J. R. Huie, M. Rabinowitz, A. M. Puccio, P. Mukherjee, M. J. Vassar, K. K. W. Wang, R. Diaz-Arrastia, D. O. Okonkwo, S. Jain, and G. T. Manley. 2019. Association between plasma GFAP concentrations and MRI abnormalities in patients with CT-negative traumatic brain injury in the TRACK-TBI cohort: A prospective multicentre study. *Lancet Neurol* 18(10):953-961.

Yuh, E. L., P. Mukherjee, H. F. Lingsma, J. K. Yue, A. R. Ferguson, W. A. Gordon, A. B. Valadka, D. M. Schnyer, D. O. Okonkwo, A. I. Maas, and G. T. Manley. 2013. Magnetic resonance imaging improves 3-month outcome prediction in mild traumatic brain injury. *Ann Neurol* 73(2):224-235.

Yuh, E. L., S. Jain, X. Sun, D. Pisica, M. H. Harris, S. R. Taylor, A. J. Markowitz, P. Mukherjee, J. Verheyden, J. T. Giacino, H. S. Levin, M. McCrea, M. B. Stein, N. R. Temkin, R. Diaz-Arrastia, C. S. Robertson, H. F. Lingsma, D. O. Okonkwo, A. I. R. Maas, G. T. Manley, O. Adeoye, N. Badjatia, K. Boase, Y. Bodien, J. D. Corrigan, K. Crawford, S. Dikmen, A. C. Duhaime, R. Ellenbogen, V. R. Feeser, A. R. Ferguson, B. Foreman, R. Gardner, E. Gaudette, L. Gonzalez, S. Gopinath, R. Gullapalli, J. C. Hemphill, G. Hotz, C. D. Keene, J. Kramer, N. Kreitzer, C. Lindsell, J. Machamer, C. Madden, A. Martin, T. McAllister, R. Merchant, L. Nelson, L. B. Ngwenya, F. Noel, A. Nolan, E. Palacios, D. Perl, M. Rabinowitz, J. Rosand, A. Sander, G. Satris, D. Schnyer, S. Seabury, A. Toga, A. Valadka, M. Vassar, and R. Zafonte. 2021. Pathological computed tomography features associated with adverse outcomes after mild traumatic brain injury: A TRACK-TBI study with external validation in CENTER-TBI. *JAMA Neurol* 78(9):1137-1148.

B

Workshop Statement of Task

A planning committee of the National Academies of Sciences, Engineering, and Medicine will organize and conduct a 1-day public workshop that brings together experts and key stakeholders to explore the needs, opportunities, gaps, and best practices surrounding data integration in learning health care systems (LHSs) for traumatic brain injury (TBI). The workshop will feature invited presentations and discussions that may be designed to:

- Explore the variables impacting how TBI patient data are collected, standardized, harmonized, accessed, and analyzed—and the implications for care and research in LHSs;
- Discuss a vision for how enhanced TBI data integration in LHSs could improve care and advance clinical and epidemiological research;
- Consider key questions and priority use cases that could be explored through integrated patient record databases and TBI registries; and
- Spotlight ongoing efforts towards building integrated research platforms and datasets for TBI.

The planning committee will develop the agenda for the workshop, select and invite speakers and discussants, and moderate the discussions. A proceedings of the presentations and discussions at the workshop will be prepared by a designated rapporteur in accordance with institutional guidelines.

C

Workshop Agenda

SESSION 1: INTRODUCTION TO THE WORKSHOP

9:00   **WELCOME AND INTRODUCTORY REMARKS**
Corinne Peek-Asa, University of California, San Diego;
Workshop Chair; Cochair, Forum on Traumatic Brain
Injury

SESSION 2: LIVED EXPERIENCES

Session Objectives:
- Underscore the challenges that arise from fragmented and uncoordinated care, and the significance of health information exchange for improving the patient experience and supporting better outcomes.
- Discussion Questions:
  - How does the fragmentation of health care records affect a patient's care, recovery, emotional well-being, and confidence in the health care system?
  - How can the voice and experiences of TBI survivors be more integrated into the development of health information exchange systems?
  - Based on the voices and experiences of TBI survivors, what recommendations should health care providers and policy makers consider to ensure that TBI patients receive cohesive and coordinated care?

87

9:10   **SESSION INTRODUCTION**
Corinne Peek-Asa, University of California, San Diego;
Workshop Chair; Cochair, Forum on Traumatic Brain Injury

9:15   **THE EFFECT OF DATA FRAGMENTATION ON THE
EXPERIENCE OF SEEKING AND RECEIVING CARE**
Lindsay Simpson, Champion Comeback Foundation

9:35   **MODERATED DISCUSSION/AUDIENCE Q&A**

**SESSION 3: INTRODUCTION TO LEARNING
HEALTH CARE SYSTEMS**

Session Objectives:
- Provide a historical context for the conceptual origin of learning health systems.
- Articulate a definition of a learning health system: What are the essential components and functions?
- Discuss the anticipated trajectory of learning health systems over the coming years, and how they can transform the overall health care landscape.
- Review how the National Academies 2022 consensus study report *Traumatic Brain Injury: A Roadmap for Accelerating Progress* provides recommendations for care and research improvements involving learning health systems.
- Discussion Questions:
  - How did the concept of a learning health care system originate; what were the primary drivers behind its inception?
  - What distinguishes a learning health care system from a traditional health care system?
  - How do these systems incorporate feedback loops to ensure continuous learning and adaptation?

9:45   **SESSION INTRODUCTION**
Odette Harris, Stanford University and VA Palo Alto Health Care System

9:50   **LEARNING HEALTH CARE SYSTEMS**
J. Michael McGinnis, National Academy of Medicine

10:10   **MODERATED DISCUSSION/AUDIENCE Q&A**

10:30   **BREAK**

SESSION 4: STAKEHOLDER PERSPECTIVES ON HOW LHSs CAN ADDRESS UNMET PRIORITIES THAT APPLY TO TBI

Session Objectives:
- Articulate the priority research questions and care needs that learning health care systems help to address.
- Explore how different partners and stakeholders support and engage with learning health care systems.
- Discussion Questions:
  - How can organizations think of an LHS more strategically and in ways that move innovation forward?
  - What infrastructure is needed to make LHS solutions more accessible?
  - What partnerships are needed to help learning health care systems implement evidence-based care delivery innovations?
  - What strategies are needed to ensure that data drives policy, and that policy drives continuous improvement in care and research systems?

10:50   **SESSION INTRODUCTION**
David Goldstein, Department of Health and Human Services

10:55   **PERSPECTIVES PANEL**
Kathryn Davidson, Centers for Medicare and Medicaid Services
Edwin Lomotan, Agency for Healthcare Research and Quality
Leora Horwitz, New York University Langone Health
Joel Scholten, Department of Veterans Affairs

11:30   **MODERATED DISCUSSION/AUDIENCE Q&A**

12:00   **LUNCH**

12:45   **HALFTIME TOUCHPOINT**

SESSION 5: ILLUSTRATIVE EXAMPLES OF LHS IN TBI

Session Objectives
- Highlight illustrative examples of how learning health systems for TBI support care delivery, improve health outcomes, and expand research opportunities.
- Discussion Questions
  - In these examples, what key achievements for research and care have been observed because of the integrated linkages between care, research, and continuous learning?
  - Across these examples of learning health care systems, what common challenges arise? What strategies are being deployed to address them?
  - What are the key lessons learned?

1:00   SESSION INTRODUCTIONS
Nsini Umoh, National Institute of Neurological Disorders and Stroke

1:05   EXEMPLARS OF LEARNING HEALTH CARE SYSTEMS IN TBI
Jennifer Bogner, Ohio State University Medical Center
Joseph Giacino, Spaulding Rehabilitation Hospital and
    Harvard Medical School
Katharine Stout, Department of Defense

1:55   MODERATED DISCUSSION/AUDIENCE Q&A

2:40   BREAK

SESSION 6: DATA CAPTURE, SURVEILLANCE, AND SUPPORTING COMMUNITY-BASED CARE

Session Objectives:
- Understand how the CDC performs data capture and surveillance to inform public health strategies and support community-based care.
- Explore how state brain health programs partner with learning health care systems to identify TBI survivors and create linkages to community services.
- Hear a high-level overview of the VA's approach to harnessing learning health care systems to enhance community care for veterans with TBI.

- Discussion Questions:
  - o What LHS-based programs exemplify a successful execution of data capture and surveillance leading to material improvements in how survivors are supported via community-based care?
  - o What are some key lessons learned?
  - o From the perspective of public health and community-based care, what do we need from learning health care systems that currently is not in place, and why is this a priority?
  - o How can data insights from such diverse entities as CDC, state departments, and VA be integrated to form a more cohesive and holistic LHS for TBI community care?

3:00   **LEARNING HEALTH CARE SYSTEMS FOR DATA CAPTURE AND SURVEILLANCE**
Kristine Yaffe, University of California, San Francisco
        (moderator)
Jill Daugherty, Centers for Disease Control and
        Prevention (virtual)

3:20   **LEARNING HEALTH CARE SYSTEMS TO SUPPORT COMMUNITY-BASED CARE**
Rebeccah Wolfkiel, National Association of State Head Injury
        Administrators (moderator)
Christiane Miller, Virginia Department for Aging and
        Rehabilitative Services

3:40   **LEARNING HEALTH CARE SYSTEMS FOR TBI IN THE DEPARTMENT OF VETERANS AFFAIRS**
Joel Scholten, Department of Veterans Affairs (moderator)
Stuart Hoffman, Department of Veterans Affairs

4:00   **MODERATED DISCUSSION/AUDIENCE Q&A**

SESSION 7: WHAT IS NEEDED FROM LHSs TO COMBAT INEQUITABLE OUTCOMES IN TBI

Session Objectives:
- Examine strategies to build and enhance the capacity of community systems to respond to and manage brain injuries, especially in geographic regions or among demographic groups that are underserved.

- Discussion Questions:
  - o What are the current gaps in TBI awareness and education for patients and providers?
  - o Why is building community capacity for TBI community care essential, and what is needed from learning health care systems to facilitate this?
  - o How might LHS-based solutions improve health outcomes for vulnerable populations of TBI-injured people—including those who are rurally located, are survivors of intimate-partner violence, or are incarcerated?
  - o For vulnerable patient populations with limited access to specialized care centers, what are the greatest barriers in the way of accessing LHS-based solutions locally?

4:20   **SESSION INTRODUCTION**
Monique Pappadis, University of Texas Medical Branch at Galveston (virtual)

4:25   **PATIENT/PROVIDER EDUCATION, RESOURCE FACILITATION, AND SYSTEMS CAPACITY BUILDING IN COMMUNITY FOR BRAIN INJURY**
Peggy Reisher, Brain Injury Alliance of Nebraska

4:40   **MODERATED DISCUSSION/AUDIENCE Q&A**

4:50   **CONCLUDING REMARKS**
Corinne Peek-Asa, University of California, San Diego; Workshop Chair; Cochair, Forum on Traumatic Brain Injury

5:00   **ADJOURN**

D

Planning Committee, Speaker, and Moderator Biographies

Jennifer Bogner, Ph.D., ABPP, is the vice chair of research and academic affairs for the Department of Physical Medicine and Rehabilitation at the Ohio State University Medical Center. She has worked within the field of traumatic brain injury rehabilitation for nearly 20 years and is a board-certified rehabilitation psychologist and professor in the Department of Physical Medicine and Rehabilitation at Ohio State. She is the coprincipal investigator of the Ohio Regional TBI Model System and is currently or has served as principal investigator or coprincipal investigator on multiple studies addressing issues associated with TBI and substance use disorders, including randomized clinical trials or interventions. Bogner has authored or coauthored more than 40 publications in professional journals and one book chapter. She has presented nationally on topics related to brain injury and serves as the associate editor of the *Journal of Head Trauma Rehabilitation.* She is a member-at-large on the board of governors of the American Congress of Rehabilitation Medicine.

Jill Daugherty, Ph.D., M.P.H., is an epidemiologist on the Traumatic Brain Injury (TBI) Team in the Division of Injury Prevention (DIP) at the Injury Center. Her work focuses on understanding the public health burden of and sociodemographic disparities in TBI. She began her career at CDC as a survey researcher at the National Center for Health Statistics (NCHS) in Hyattsville, Maryland, working on the National Survey of Family Growth. After 3 years at NCHS she transferred to DIP in Atlanta, Georgia. Daugherty received a bachelor of science degree in biobehavioral health from Penn State University and a master of public health and doctorate in sociology from Emory University. She has authored or coauthored more than 20 peer-reviewed journal articles and government reports.

Kathryn Davidson, LCSW, is the director of the learning and diffusion group at the Center for Medicare and Medicaid Innovation (CMMI), within the Centers for Medicare & Medicaid Services (CMS). In this role, Davidson leads CMMI's team, focused on accelerating health care system transformation by using improvement science within and across models, as well as leading the multipayer alignment strategy for CMMI through the Healthcare Payment Learning and Action Network (HCP-LAN). Prior to joining CMS, Davidson led Policy and Practice Improvement efforts at the National Council for Mental Wellbeing, where she managed payment reform, quality improvement, and workforce development initiatives in mental health and addiction prevention, treatment, and recovery organizations and provided training and technical assistance to human services organizations, counties, and states. Davidson began her career in health care as a social worker researching, testing, and scaling interventions in community-based settings. She has an M.S.W. from Fordham University and a B.A. from Loyola College in Maryland.

Joseph T. Giacino, Ph.D., is the director of rehabilitation neuropsychology at Spaulding Rehabilitation Hospital, consulting neuropsychologist in the Department of Psychiatry at Massachusetts General Hospital, and professor of physical medicine and rehabilitation at Harvard Medical School. Giacino's clinical and research activities are centered on the development and application of novel assessment and treatment methods for individuals with severe acquired brain injury and disorders of consciousness (DOC). He served as cochair of the Aspen Workgroup, responsible for developing the diagnostic criteria for the minimally conscious state and was colead author of the Mohonk Report, a congressionally sponsored initiative to establish recommendations for lifelong care of patients with DOC. He currently chairs the VS/MCS Guideline Development Panel of the American Academy of Neurology, which is responsible for revising existing guidelines for the management of patients with DOC. He is principle investigator on a project funded by the National Institute on Disability and Rehabilitation Research (NIDRR) to develop novel fMRI paradigms to assess the integrity of language and visual processing networks in patients with DOC. He serves as project director of a 12-site NIDRR-funded clinical trial of amantadine hydrochloride (AH) to determine whether AH facilitates functional recovery in patients with prolonged DOC. He also served as Co-PI of an FDA-approved pilot study of deep brain stimulation aimed at promoting recovery of speech and motor functions in patients with chronic post-traumatic minimally conscious state.

David Goldstein, M.S. OTR/L, serves as a senior advisor within the Immediate Office of the Assistant Secretary for Health (OASH) at the Department of Health and Human Services (HHS). Within this role, Goldstein advises the deputy assistant secretary for science and medicine as well as the chief medical officer regarding program priorities covering the full range of public health activities within the HHS Office of the Assistant Secretary for Health with a focus on those relating to public health innovation, clinical care delivery, health care payment and reimbursement policy, and the intersection of clinical care delivery and population health safety and preparedness. The Office of the Assistant Secretary for Health oversees HHS key public health offices and programs, several presidential and secretarial advisory committees, 10 regional public health offices across the nation, the Office of the Surgeon General, and the U.S. Public Health Service Commissioned Corps. Prior to his arrival at HHS, Goldstein served as a public health adviser at the Center for Medicare and Medicaid Innovation and as behavioral health lead for emerging model topics focused on behavioral health care delivery system transformation for those with unmet mental health and substance use disorder diagnoses and care needs. He is a licensed occupational therapist and prior to his transition into health policy was in clinical practice at the University of California, San Diego, Medical Center, delivering hospital-based specialty rehabilitation care to patients with chronic complex care needs. His background also includes work as a federal health care management consultant supporting the Navy Bureau of Medicine's Directorate of Healthcare Business in San Diego, focused on the development of a patient-centered medical home model for Navy (TRI-CARE) beneficiaries, as well as advisory work with the Camden Coalition of Healthcare Providers on their academic and practice-based complex care collaboratives. Goldstein received his Master of Science in Occupational Therapy from Thomas Jefferson University.

Odette Harris, M.D., M.P.H., is the Paralyzed Veterans of America, Endowed Professor of Spinal Cord Injury Medicine; a professor of neurosurgery; and the vice chair, diversity, and director of brain injury for Stanford. She is the Deputy Chief of Staff, Rehabilitation, at the Veterans Affairs Palo Alto Health Care System, overseeing the TBI/Polytrauma System of Care, Spinal Cord Injury, Blind Rehabilitation Services, Recreational Therapy, and Physical Medicine & Rehabilitation. Harris graduated from Dartmouth College and received her M.D. from Stanford University School of Medicine. She did her internship and residency at Stanford and earned a Master of Public Health, Epidemiology, from the University of California, Berkeley. Dr. Harris has authored numerous articles and books and is a member of several editorial boards and national committees, including as the associate editor for *Neurosurgery* and as an appointed member, National Football League

(NFL) Head, Neck and Spine Committee. She also serves on several boards including the Defense Health Board's (DHB) Trauma and Injury Subcommittee and is a Trustee of Dartmouth College. She has won numerous awards: appointed a Fellow of the Aspen Global Leadership Network in 2018, recognized in 2019 by *Forbes* and *Ebony Magazine* Power 100 List Award as one of 100 most influential African Americans, and received the National Medical Fellowships Award for Excellence in Academic Medicine. In 2021 she received the Stanford RISE Award. In 2022 Harris was recognized by Stanford University as one of Stanford's 13 women's history makers. Harris' Endowed Professorship further distinguishes her as the first woman in neurosurgery at Stanford to receive this honor.

Stuart Hoffman, Ph.D., is the senior health science officer for TBI for the Office of Research and Development (ORD), Veterans Health Administration, Department of Veteran Affairs (VA). Dr. Hoffman assumed his role in January 2020. He is responsible for supporting the National Research Action Plan activities; serving as VA lead for the joint VA/Department of Defense Long-term Impact of Military-relevant Brain Injury Consortium (LIMBIC); providing overall direction, program planning, development and implementation for ORD TBI research; coordinating with ORD leads and federal partners in other high-priority nationwide efforts in brain health; promoting data sharing in TBI research; and expanding the clinical trials network nationally to improve TBI treatments and diagnostics for veterans. Hoffman joined the Rehabilitation Research and Development Service in ORD in February 2010 where he served as the scientific program manager for brain health and injury. His accomplishments included doubling the RRD TBI portfolio, creating a special emphasis area for proposals investigating the long-term effects of prescribed and nonprescribed drugs on outcome from TBI, and oversight of two successful research centers. Hoffman has previously coordinated TBI research initiatives such as the Chronic Effects of Neurotrauma Consortium Government Steering Committee and is the VA representative on the National Academies of Sciences, Engineering, and Medicine Forum on Neuroscience and Nervous System Disorders. In 2015, he chaired the Scientific Planning Committee for the second VA TBI State of the Art (SOTA) Conference. Hoffman received his Ph.D. in behavioral and molecular neuroscience at Rutgers University in 1995 and completed his postdoctoral training in pharmacology at Virginia Commonwealth University in 1997. Hoffman was a full-time Emory University faculty member from 1998 to 2006. Immediately prior to joining the VA in 2010, Hoffman was the Research Director for the Defense and Veterans Brain Injury Center in Johnstown, Pennsylvania. He has authored more than 50 peer-reviewed publications and has more than 35 years of translational neuroscience research experience focused on TBI therapeutics.

Leora Horwitz, M.D., is a general internist who studied social science as an undergraduate and is now a clinician researcher focused on quality and safety in health care. In particular, she focuses on systems and practices intended to bridge gaps or discontinuities in care. She has studied shift-to-shift transfers among physicians and among nurses, transfers from the emergency department to inpatient units, and the transition from the hospital to home. She is currently adjunct faculty at Yale; her primary work is at NYU Langone Health, where she directs the Center for Healthcare Innovation and Delivery Science and the Division of Health Care Delivery Science in the Department of Population Health. Her current work is focused primarily on developing a learning health system through innovations in clinical delivery and in data capture and analysis.

Michael F. Huerta, Ph.D., is acting deputy director for operations and innovation at the National Library of Medicine (NLM). In this role, he develops frameworks and models for innovation and new growth opportunities. Huerta also provides administrative oversight for the overall NLM research portfolio, serves as NLM chief diversity officer, and provides senior executive support to NLM's division and office directors. Huerta has spent more than 30 years at NIH and has made major contributions to the development and implementation of open science, as well as large-scale, open, digital biomedical research and technology initiatives. Most recently, he directed the NLM Office of Strategic Initiatives and served as associate director of NLM for Strategy to identify, implement, and assess strategic directions of NLM. Throughout his tenure at NIH, Huerta has led many NIH research initiatives, including the NIH Human Connectome Project, the National Database for Autism Research, and the U.S. Human Brain Project, which was key in creating and establishing the field of neuroinformatics. He chairs several committees across NIH and NLM to help realize the promise of data science and open science for biomedicine. Huerta's research background is in systems neuroscience; his undergraduate and doctoral work was completed at the University of Wisconsin at Madison, he was an NIH postdoctoral fellow at Vanderbilt University, and he was on the faculty of the University of Connecticut Health Center before joining NIH's National Institute of Mental Health in 1991 and moving to the National Library of Medicine in 2011.

Edwin Lomotan, M.D., FAMIA, serves as senior advisor for clinical informatics in the Center for Evidence and Practice Improvement at the Agency for Healthcare Research and Quality (AHRQ). He currently leads AHRQ's clinical decision support (CDS) initiative, which aims to advance evidence into practice through CDS and to make CDS more shareable, standards-based, and publicly available. Lomotan is board certified in clinical informatics and received his medical degree from the University of Pittsburgh. He completed his pediatrics residency and informatics fellowship at Yale University. He also spent several years in community pediatric practice in Connecticut before joining federal service in 2010.

J. Michael McGinnis, M.D., is a physician and epidemiologist who lives and works in Washington, DC. Through his scholarly contributions, government service, and work in philanthropy, he has been a long-time contributor to national and global leadership in population health and medicine. Currently the Leonard D. Schaefer executive officer of the National Academy of Medicine (NAM), NAM senior scholar, and executive director of the NAM Leadership Consortium, previously he was founding director, respectively, of the Robert Wood Johnson Foundation's (RWJF) Health Group, the World Health Organization's Office for Health Reconstruction in Bosnia, and the Department of Health and Human Services (HHS) federal Office of Disease Prevention and Health Promotion, and federal Office of Research Integrity (interim). At HHS, he held appointments as assistant surgeon general and deputy assistant secretary for health, with continuous policy leadership responsibility for federal activities in disease prevention and health promotion from 1977 to 1995, a tenure unusual for political and policy posts.

Christiane Miller, M.B.A., is the director of Virginia's Department for Aging and Rehabilitative Services (DARS) Brain Injury Services Coordination Unit. Prior to this position she spent 35 years developing housing and supportive services for people with disabilities, creating livable communities for older adults, and directing a free clinic for uninsured adults. As part of her role at DARS, Miller oversees the Commonwealth Neurotrauma Initiative, a trust fund that makes grants to Virginia-based researchers and organizations improving services for individuals living with spinal cord injuries and traumatic brain injuries. Working with Virginia's TBI Model Systems, the Brain Injury Association of Virginia, NASHIA, and other community partners, she is leading the effort develop a Data Plan for Brain Injury across systems and state agencies. Miller received her B.S. in psychology at Mary Washington College and a master's in business administration at Averett University.

Monique R. Pappadis, M.Ed., Ph.D., is a tenured associate professor in the Department of Population Health and Health Disparities at the University of Texas Medical Branch (UTMB) at Galveston. She is a fellow of the Sealy Center on Aging, and currently the Diversity, Equity, Inclusion and Accessibility (DEIA) lead for the CTSA Program Steering Committee Task Force/ Institute for Translational Sciences. Pappadis is also an investigator and the director of dissemination and cultural humility at TIRR Memorial Hermann's Brain Injury Research Center in Houston, Texas. Her research aims to improve rehabilitation outcomes and decrease ethnic minority health disparities, particularly among persons with traumatic brain injury (TBI) or stroke, as well as improve care transitions and continuity of care following acute and postacute care. Her recent work aims to improve screening for elder mistreatment with emphasis on vulnerable, older adults with mild cognitive impairment or Alzheimer's disease and related dementias, as well as the intersection between elder mistreatment and TBI. She has a continued interest in minority aging, gender/sex disparities in rehabilitation, health literacy of patients and caregivers, and psychosocial adjustment to disability. She is a member of the Academy of Certified Brain Injury Specialists' (ACBIS) Board of Governors for the Brain Injury Association of American and member of the Pink Concussions Professional Advisory Board. Pappadis was recently named a fellow of the American Congress of Rehabilitation Medicine (ACRM) for her outstanding record of professional service to ACRM and for the nationally significant contributions she has made to the field of medical rehabilitation.

Corinne Peek-Asa, Ph.D., M.P.H., is the vice chancellor for research and professor with distinction of epidemiology at UC San Diego. She is an elected member of the National Academy of Medicine and served as a member of the National Academies Committee on Accelerating Progress in Traumatic Brain Injury and Care and the Global Violence Forum. Prior to joining UC San Diego, she was the associate dean for research for the University of Iowa College of Public Health and the William G. Battershell distinguished professor. Peek-Asa is a leading epidemiologist in traumatic injury and violence prevention. Peek-Asa's work has addressed the full spectrum of traumatic brain injuries from surveillance to prevention among a variety of populations. Peek-Asa has led international traumatic brain injury research, including a role as principal investigator on NIH FIC and NINDS projects that have established prospective traumatic brain injury registries in four countries. She has conducted research on data systems to identify TBI, the effect of gender on TBI outcomes, predictors of outcomes based on injury type and severity, the effect of trauma systems on TBI patients reaching definitive care, and she has evaluated numerous TBI prevention strategies such as motorcycle helmet legislation.

Peggy Reisher, M.S.W., is executive director of the Brain Injury Alliance of Nebraska (BIA-NE). Reisher has worked in the field of brain injury for over 25 years. She helped establish the BIA-NE in 2009 and became its executive director in July 2013, previously serving as the director of programs and services. Reisher has a master's degree in social work and worked 14 years on the traumatic brain injury unit at Madonna Rehabilitation Hospital in

Lincoln, Nebraska, where she helped patients and families identify community resources upon discharge from the hospital. Reisher is currently the president of the United States Brain Injury Alliance and is on the Munroe Meyer Institute board of directors.

Joel Scholten, M.D., is executive director of Physical Medicine & Rehabilitation at the Department of Veterans Affairs (VA) and also serves as the associate chief of staff for rehabilitation services at the Washington, DC, VA Medical Center. His research interests include traumatic brain injury, polytrauma, and pain. He received his medical degree at the University of South Dakota and completed his residency in physical medicine and rehabilitation at Eastern Virginia Graduate School of Medicine. Scholten joined VA in 1998 as medical director of the Brain Injury Rehabilitation program at the Tampa VA before transferring to the Washington, DC, VA Medical Center in 2009.

Lindsay Simpson is an Emmy-award-winning sports reporter and former soccer goalkeeper at the University of Maryland. After suffering a significant traumatic brain injury in 2018 that nearly took her life, she has turned her attention to advocating for brain trauma awareness and support. Her own medical battle has been long and arduous, and as she continues to adapt to her "new normal" she uses her experiences to help others through their own brain trauma recovery. She has launched a nonprofit, the Champion Comeback Foundation, which provides resources for those recovering from brain injuries, mentorship for athletes and former athletes who have experienced brain trauma, and a support network for their caregivers.

Katharine Stout, D.P.T., M.B.A., PT, NCS, is assistant branch chief at the Department of Defense Traumatic Brain Injury Center of Excellence (TBI-CoE). She received her doctorate in physical therapy from Northeastern University and her master's in business administration with a concentration in health care administration from the University of Scranton. She is a board-certified neurological specialist by the American Board of Physical Therapy Specialties. For the last 12 years she has worked in TBI and military medicine in a variety of roles including direct clinical care, research portfolio management, and program management. In addition to her work with the military, she is adjunct faculty at the University of Maryland School of Medicine and served a 4-year term as a board member for the Maryland Board of Physical Therapy Examiners 2013–2017. She has authored several publications and a book chapter.

Nsini Umoh, Ph.D., is a program director in the Repair and Plasticity Cluster in the Division of Neuroscience. Umoh received her Ph.D. at Howard University in the Department of Physiology and Biophysics and did postdoctoral training in extremity trauma at Yale University and the U.S. Army Institute of Surgical Research. Before joining NINDS, she served as a scientific program manager at the Department of Veterans Affairs (VA) Office of Research & Development. While at VA, she managed research related to traumatic brain injury, women's health, and health equity. Before joining VA, Umoh spent 3 years as a portfolio manager at the Department of Defense (DoD) Medical Research and Development Command (MRDC) headquartered in Frederick, Maryland. While at MRDC, she worked with the Combat Casualty Care Research Program (CCCRP) to manage research related to the early management of combat-related neurotrauma on the battlefield. As a NINDS TBI program director, Umoh manages a broad research portfolio including translational and clinical research, serves as codirector of the Federal Interagency TBI Research informatics platform, and works with national and international partners.

Rebeccah Wolfkiel, M.P.P., joined NASHIA as executive director in January 2018. She brings 15 years of experience in promoting policies that provide resources for individuals with brain injury and their families. In her role as executive director, Wolfkiel is committed to representing the interests of state governments and supporting the unique and integral role they play within the service delivery system. Wolfkiel also worked with former Pennsylvania governor, Tom Ridge, at the Ridge Policy Group, for 10 years, where she formerly represented NASHIA as a government affairs advisor. She played an integral role in the successful reauthorization of the Traumatic Brain Injury in 2014, paving the way for the federal TBI program's move to the Administration for Community Living. Prior to her time at the Ridge Policy Group, Rebeccah worked on Capitol Hill for over 6 years where she served as legislative director to Congressman Todd R. Platts, cochair of the Traumatic Brain Injury Taskforce. Managing the congressman's legislative agenda, she learned how to effectively navigate the lawmaking process and develop successful strategies. During her tenure on the Hill, Rebeccah became keenly aware of the importance of bipartisanship and developed strong congressional relationships with Republicans and Democrats alike. She often bridged partisan gaps and facilitated communication between contrasting viewpoints. Wolfkiel received a Bachelor of Arts from Dickinson College in Carlisle, Pennsylvania, and a Master of Public Policy from George Mason University in Arlington, Virginia.

Kristine Yaffe, M.D., is the Scola Endowed chair and vice chair, professor of psychiatry, neurology, and epidemiology, and director of the Center for Population Brain Health at the University of California, San Francisco. Yaffe is dually trained in neurology and psychiatry and completed postdoctoral training in epidemiology and geriatric psychiatry, all at UCSF. In addition to her positions at UCSF, Yaffe is the chief of neuropsychiatry and the director of the Memory Evaluation Clinic at the San Francisco Veterans Affairs Health Care System. In her research, clinical work, and mentoring, she has worked towards improving the care of patients with cognitive disorders and other geriatric neuropsychiatric conditions. Yaffe is an internationally recognized expert in the epidemiology of dementia and cognitive aging and the foremost leader in identifying modifiable risk factors for dementia. Her research, currently supported by over a dozen NIH, Department of Defense, VA, and foundation grants, bridges the fields of neurology, psychiatry, and epidemiology. Yaffe was the first to determine that potentially 30 percent of dementia risk is preventable. She pioneered early investigations on the roles of estrogen, physical activity, and cardiovascular factors in dementia risk, and more recently, her research group has led work on the connections between cognitive aging and sleep disorders, traumatic brain injury, and life-course exposures. With over 600 peer-reviewed articles dedicated to improving population brain health (H-index = 152 and recognized by Clarivate Analytics as one of the most highly cited researchers in her field), her work has formed the cornerstone for dementia prevention trials worldwide. In recognition of these accomplishments, Yaffe received the Potamkin Prize for Alzheimer's Research in 2017 and was elected to the National Academy of Medicine in 2019.